Study Guide for

Nursing Research: Methods and Critical Appraisal for Evidence-Based Practice

Seventh Edition

Carey A. Berry, MS, BSN, RN
Clinical Nurse
Gastrointestinal Surgical Oncology
M.D. Anderson Cancer Center
The University of Texas
Houston, Texas

Jennifer Yost, PhD, RN
Post-Doctoral Student
McMaster University School of Nursing
Hamilton, Ontario
Canada

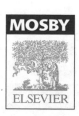

MOSBY

ELSEVIER

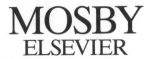

3251 Riverport Lane
St. Louis, Missouri 63043

Study Guide for Nursing Research: Methods and Critical Appraisal for
Evidence-Based Practice, Seventh Edition

978-0-323-05746-2

Notice

Knowledge and best practice in this field are constantly changing. As new research and experience broaden our knowledge, changes in practice, treatment and drug therapy may become necessary or appropriate. Readers are advised to check the most current information provided (i) on procedures featured or (ii) by the manufacturer of each product to be administered, to verify the recommended dose or formula, the method and duration of administration, and contraindications. It is the responsibility of the practitioner, relying on their own experience and knowledge of the patient, to make diagnoses, to determine dosages and the best treatment for each individual patient, and to take all appropriate safety precautions. To the fullest extent of the law, neither the Publisher nor the authors assume any liability for any injury and/or damage to persons or property arising out of or related to any use of the material contained in this book.

Previous editions copyrighted 2006, 2003, 1998

International Standard Book Number: 978-0-323-05746-2

Acquisitions Editor: Maureen Iannuzzi
Editorial Assistant: Julia Curcio
Publishing Services Manager: Jeffrey Patterson
Project Manager: Mary G. Stueck
Design Direction: Teresa McBryan

Printed in the United States of America

Last digit is the print number: 9 8 7 6 5 4 3 2

Introduction

Information bombards us! The student lament used to be "I can't find any information on X." Now the cry is "What do I do with all of the information on X?" The focus shifts from finding information to thinking about how to use and filter information. What information is worth keeping? What should be discarded? What is useful to clinical practice? What is fluff? Where are the gaps?

Thinking about the links between information and practice is critical to the improvement of the nursing care we deliver. As each of us strengthens our individual understanding of the links between interventions and outcomes, we move nursing's collective practice closer to being truly evidence-based. We can "know" what intervention works best in what situation.

"Helping people get better safely and efficiently" begins with thinking. Our intent is that the activities in the Study Guide will help you strengthen your skills in thinking about information found in the literature. The activities are designed to assist you in evaluating the research you read so you are prepared to undertake the critical analysis of research studies. As you practice the appraisal skills addressed in this Study Guide, you will be strengthening your ability to make evidence-based practice decisions grounded in theory and research.

What an incredible time to be a nurse!

General Directions

1. We recommend that you read the textbook chapter first, then complete the Study Guide activities for that chapter.

2. Complete each chapter and the activities in that chapter. This Study Guide is designed so that you build on the knowledge gained in Chapter 1 to complete the activities in Chapter 2, and so forth. The activities are designed to give you the opportunity to apply the knowledge learned in the textbook and actually use this knowledge to solve problems, thereby gaining increased confidence that comes only from working through each chapter.

3. Follow the specific directions that precede each activity. Be certain that you have the resources needed to complete the activity before you begin.

4. Do the posttest after all of the chapter's activities have been completed. The answers for the posttest items can be found in the answer key. If you answer 85% of the questions correctly, be confident that you have grasped the essential material presented in the chapter.

5. Clarify any questions, confusion, or concerns you may have with your instructor.

ACTIVITY ANSWERS ARE IN THE BACK OF THIS BOOK

Answers in a workbook such as this do not follow a formula like answers in a math book. Many times you are asked to make a judgment about a particular problem. If your judgment differs from that of the authors, review the criteria that you used to make your decision. Determine if you followed a logical progression of steps to reach your conclusion. If not, rework the activity. If the process you followed appears logical, and your answer remains different, remember that even experts may disagree on many of the judgment calls in nursing research. There will continue to be many "gray areas." If you average an 85% agreement with the authors, you can be sure that you are on the right track and should feel very confident about your level of expertise.

Carey A. Berry, MS, BSN, RN

Jennifer Yost, PhD, RN

Contents

1

Integrating the Processes of Research and Evidence-Based Practice

INTRODUCTION

One goal of this chapter in the study guide is to assist you in reviewing the material presented in Chapter 1 of the text written by LoBiondo-Wood and Haber. A second and more fundamental goal is to provide you with an opportunity to begin practicing the role of a critical consumer of research. Succeeding chapters in this workbook fine-tune your ability to evaluate research studies critically.

LEARNING OUTCOMES

On completion of this chapter, the student should be able to do the following:

- State the significance of research to evidence-based nursing practice.
- Identify the role of the consumer of nursing research.
- Define *evidence-based practice.*
- Discuss evidence-based decision making.
- Explain the difference between quantitative and qualitative research.
- Explain the difference among types of systematic reviews: integrative review, meta-analysis, and meta-synthesis.
- Identify the importance of critical thinking and critical reading skills for critical appraisal of research studies.
- Discuss the format and style of research reports/articles.
- Discuss how to use a quantitative evidence hierarchy when critically appraising research studies.

Activity 1

Match the term in Column B with the appropriate phrase in Column A. Each term will be used only once. This may be a good time to review the glossary.

	Column A		Column B
1. _____	Systematic inquiry into possible relationships among particular phenomena	a.	Critique
2. _____	One who reads critically and applies research findings in nursing practice	b.	Consumer
		c.	Research
3. _____	Synthesis and review of the literature on a specific topic without statistical analysis	d.	Integrative review
		e.	Systematic review
4. _____	Critically evaluates a research report's content based on a set of criteria to evaluate the scientific merit for application	f.	Evidence-based practice
		g.	Research utilization
5. _____	Implementation of a scientifically sound research-based innovation into clinical practice	h.	Clinical guidelines
6. _____	Summary and assessment of a group of quantitative studies that used similar designs to study a focused clinical question		
7. _____	Clinical practice based upon the collection, interpretation, and integration of expert knowledge, research-derived evidence, and patient preferences		
8. _____	Practice statements systematically developed on a national level to assist clinicians make health care decisions about specific conditions or situations		

Activity 2

Match the term in Column B with the appropriate phrase in Column A. Terms from Column B will be used more than once.

	Column A		Column B
1. _____	Systematic investigation of nursing phenomena	a.	Research
2. _____	Follows scientific method	b.	Evidence-based practice
3. _____	Collection, interpretation, and integration of research evidence combined with clinical experience and patient preference		
4. _____	Critical appraisal of completed studies on clinical question		
5. _____	May be quantitative or qualitative		

Activity 3

Match the term in Column B with the appropriate phrase in Column A. Terms from Column B will be used more than once.

	Column A	**Column B**
1. _____	To get a general sense of the material	a. Critical thinking
2. _____	Clarify unfamiliar terms with text	b. Critical reading
3. _____	Using constructive skepticism	
4. _____	Question assumptions	
5. _____	Rational examination of ideas	
6. _____	Thinking about your own thinking	
7. _____	Allows assessment of study validity	

Activity 4

Complete each item with the appropriate word or phrase from the text.

1. Critical thinking is the examination of _____, _____, _____, _____, _____, _____, and _____.

2. Paul and Elder (2008) state that critical reading is defined as "an (active; passive), intellectually engaging process in which the reader participates in an (inner; outer) dialogue with (the writer, themselves)."

3. What is the minimum number of readings of a research article recommended in the text? _____

4. Place the four stages of critical reading in order of levels of understanding:

   _____

   _____

   _____

   _____

5. Key variables, new terms, and steps of the research process should be understood following a(n) _____ understanding of a research article.

6. With _____ understanding of a research article, you should be able to state the main idea or study intent in one or two sentences.

7. Analysis of an article will allow understanding of the _____ of a study; synthesis will allow an understanding of the _____ article and all steps in the research process.

Activity 5

Determine whether the article in Appendix B of the text (Jones, Renger, & Kang, 2007) is a quantitative or qualitative study. Use the following points to determine if the study you are reading is of a quantitative design. First answer *yes* or *no* for each item, and then summarize your thoughts in a paragraph.

1.	Hypotheses are stated or implied in the article.	Yes	No
2.	The terms *treatment or intervention* and *control or comparison group* appear.	Yes	No
3.	The terms *survey, correlational,* or *ex post facto* are used. (*Note:* Read the glossary definitions for help in answering this question.)	Yes	No
4.	The terms *random* or *convenience* are mentioned in relation to the sample.	Yes	No
5.	Variables are measured by instruments or tools.	Yes	No
6.	Reliability and validity of instruments are discussed.	Yes	No
7.	Statistical analyses are used.	Yes	No

Summary:

Activity 6

Now that you have read the chapter, answer the following questions in your own words in a way that is meaningful to you.

1. Why is knowing about nursing research important?

2. How will nurses produce depth in nursing science?

3. If you were asked to give testimony about your practice to the local city council, state assembly, or senate, what research information would you like to have to assist you in presenting the testimony?

Activity 7: Web-Based Activity

Go to the website www.ahrq.gov/about/nursing/ and read the following:

a. About nurses at AHRQ
b. Clinical Information (under main menu)
c. Future Directions in Primary Care Research: New Special Issues for Nurses (found under Tools and Resources)
d. Under the title "Research Findings," choose a research activity and read the report.

Activity 8: Evidence-Based Practice Activity

1. Using appendix A (Meneses, McNees, Loerzel, et al., 2007) and Appendix D (Landreneau & Ward-Smith, 2007) list the type of article (quantitative, qualitative) and the level of evidence (using Figure 1-1).

   a. Meneses et al.: _____, _____

   b. Landreneau & Ward Smith: _____, _____

2. Find a research article in your area of practice. Determine the level of evidence for the article.

POSTTEST

1. In analyzing research articles it is important to remember that the researcher may (omit; vary) the steps slightly, but that the steps must still be systematically addressed.

2. To critically read a research study, the reader must have skilled reading, writing, and reasoning abilities. Use these abilities to read the following abstract, and then identify concepts, clarify any unfamiliar concepts or terms, and question any assumptions or rationales presented.

   In this study we examined pain and disability in 115 community-dwelling, urban, older adults. . . . Sixty percent of the sample reported experiencing pain. In this sample, 66 (57.4%) participants reported having physical limitations in at least one item on the physical mobility subscale of the SIP. Pain was significantly associated with greater functional disability in both physical and social functional domains, highlighting the important real-world consequences of living with pain. Pain is a common problem, and its high prevalence (60%) in this sample of individuals over 60 years of age is consistent with epidemiological studies of pain. . . . Pain was significantly associated with greater functional disability in both physical and social functional domains, highlighting the important real-world consequences of living with pain. Contrary to previous research, race was not related to pain in this sample (Horgas, Yoon, Nichols, & Marsiske, 2008).

   a. Identify concepts.

    b.   List any unfamiliar concepts or terms that you would need to clarify.

    c.   What assumptions or rationales would you question?

3.   Quantitative and qualitative articles vary a great deal in format and style when they appear in journals. The following statements will focus your attention on these differences and help you to distinguish between the two major types of research. Answer the following questions by inserting the correct term from the list provided. Not all terms will be used.

      Used   Conducted
      Generate hypotheses   Test a hypothesis
      Statistical tests   Analyze themes or concepts

    a.   The primary difference between the two is that the qualitative study does not
_____ but may _____.

    b.   An additional major difference is in the way the literature reviews are
_____ and _____ in the study.

REFERENCES

Horgas AL, Yoon SL, Nichols AL, et al.: The relationship between pain and functional disability in black and white older adults, *Res Nurs Health* 31(4):341-354, 2008.

Jones EG, Renger R, Kang Y: Self-efficacy for health-related behaviors among deaf adults, *Res Nurs Health* 30:185-192, 2007.

Landreneau KJ, Ward-Smith P: Perceptions of adult patients on hemodialysis concerning choice among renal replacement therapies, *Nephrol Nurs* 34(5):513-519, 525, 2007.

Meneses DK, McNees P, Loerzel W, et al.: Transition from treatment to survivorship: Effects of a psychoeducational intervention on quality of life in breast cancer survivors, *Oncol Nurs Forum* 34:1007-1016, 2007.

Paul R, Elder L: The miniature guide to critical thinking: Concepts and tools, Dillon Beach, CA, 2008, Foundation for Critical Thinking.

U.S. Department of Health and Human Services: Agency for Healthcare Research and Quality. Retrieved August 19, 2009, from www.ahcpr.gov/.

2

Research Questions, Hypotheses, and Clinical Questions

INTRODUCTION

This chapter focuses on identifying research questions, hypotheses, and clinical questions. If developed correctly, research questions can be very helpful to you as a research consumer because they concisely describe the essence of the research study. Research questions present the idea that is to be examined in the study. Hypotheses, which extend from the literature review and research questions, are predictions that provide a vehicle for testing the relationships between variables. For the nurse who considers using the results of a given study in practice, the two primary concerns are to locate and critique the research question and hypotheses. The research question or hypotheses provide the most succinct link between the underlying theoretical base and guide the design of the research study. Although similar to research questions, clinical questions are developed by the nurse to provide answers to clinical situations. Clinical questions, framed using the PICO format, are the basis for searching the literature to identify the best available evidence for clinical situations.

LEARNING OUTCOMES

On completion of this chapter, the student should be able to do the following:

- Describe how the research question and hypothesis relate to the other components of the research process.
- Describe the process of identifying and refining a research question.
- Identify the criteria for determining the significance of a research question.
- Discuss the purpose of developing a clinical question.
- Discuss the appropriate use of the purpose, aim, or objective of a research study.
- Discuss how the purpose, research question, and hypothesis suggest the level of evidence to be obtained from the findings of a research study.
- Describe the advantages and disadvantages of directional and nondirectional hypotheses.
- Compare and contrast the use of statistical versus research hypotheses.
- Discuss the appropriate use of research questions versus hypotheses in a research study.
- Discuss the differences between a research question and a clinical question in relation to evidence-based practice.
- Identify the criteria used for critiquing a research question and hypothesis.
- Apply the critiquing criteria to the evaluation of a research question and hypothesis in a research report.

Activity 1

Match the terms in Column B to the appropriate phrase in Column A. Not all terms from Column B will be used.

<table>
<tr><td colspan="2" align="center">**Column A**</td><td align="center">**Column B**</td></tr>
<tr><td>1. _____</td><td>Statement about the relationship between two or more variables</td><td>a. Testability
b. Independent variable</td></tr>
<tr><td>2. _____</td><td>The variable that has the presumed effect on the second variable</td><td>c. Variables
d. Dependent variable</td></tr>
<tr><td>3. _____</td><td>The nonmanipulated variable that the researcher is interested in understanding, explaining, or predicting</td><td>e. Research question
f. Hypothesis</td></tr>
<tr><td>4. _____</td><td>A property of the research question that expresses a relationship between variables implying that it is measurable by either qualitative or quantitative methods</td><td></td></tr>
<tr><td>5. _____</td><td>The concepts or properties that are operationalized and studied</td><td></td></tr>
<tr><td>6. _____</td><td>Statement that presents the idea(s) to be examined in the study</td><td></td></tr>
</table>

Activity 2

A good research question exhibits three characteristics. Critique the research questions below to determine if each of the three criteria is present. Following each problem statement is a list representing the three criteria (a, b, and c). Circle *yes* or *no* to indicate whether each criterion is met.

The research question:

a. Clearly identifies the variable(s) under consideration
b. Specifies the population being studied
c. Implies the possibility of empirical testing

1. The purpose of this study was to compare substance involvement among adolescent smokers in a psychiatric inpatient facility who had received either a motivational interviewing intervention or brief advice for smoking cessation (Brown et al., 2009).

Criterion a: Yes   No

Criterion b: Yes   No

Criterion c: Yes   No

2. The purpose of this study was to determine if a predictive relationship exists between critical thinking and success in nursing. Success in nursing was defined as passing the NCLEX-RN® on the first attempt (Shirrell, 2008).

   Criterion a: Yes   No

   Criterion b: Yes   No

   Criterion c: Yes   No

3. The purpose of this study was to describe the experience of the use of community services, including benefits and barriers, by family caregivers of relatives with Alzheimer's disease or a related disorder (Winslow, 2003).

   Criterion a: Yes   No

   Criterion b: Yes   No

   Criterion c: Yes   No

4. The purpose of this study was to assess self-perception of body weight among a selected sample of Taipei, Taiwan, high school students and other weight-related factors such as weight management practices, weight management goal, weight satisfaction, perception of physical attractiveness, and normative perceptions of schoolmates regarding weight loss (Page, Lee, & Miao, 2005).

   Criterion a: Yes   No

   Criterion b: Yes   No

   Criterion c: Yes   No

5. The aim of this study was to explore cancer patients' experiences of nursing pain management during hospitalization for cancer treatment (Rustøen, Gaardsrud, Leegaard, & Wahl, 2009).

   Criterion a: Yes   No

   Criterion b: Yes   No

   Criterion c: Yes   No

Activity 3

Research questions are used to guide all types of research studies. Identify whether you would expect a quantitative or qualitative research study design from the research questions in Activity 2.

Key:

   a.   Quantitative
   b.   Qualitative

1. _____   The purpose of this study was to compare substance involvement among adolescent smokers in a psychiatric inpatient facility who had received either a motivational interviewing intervention or brief advice for smoking cessation (Brown et al., 2009).

2. _____ The purpose of this study was to determine if a predictive relationship exists between critical thinking and success in nursing. Success in nursing was defined as passing the NCLEX-RN® on the first attempt (Shirrell, 2008).

3. _____ The purpose of this study was to describe the experience of the use of community services, including benefits and barriers, by family caregivers of relatives with Alzheimer's disease or a related disorder (Winslow, 2003).

4. _____ The purpose of this study was to assess self-perception of body weight among a selected sample of Taipei, Taiwan, high school students and other weight-related factors such as weight management practices, weight management goal, weight satisfaction, perception of physical attractiveness, and normative perceptions of schoolmates regarding weight loss (Page, Lee, & Miao, 2005).

5. _____ The aim of this study was to explore cancer patients' experiences of nursing pain management during hospitalization for cancer treatment (Rustøen, Gaardsrud, Leegaard, & Wahl, 2009).

Activity 4

The ability to distinguish between independent and dependent variables is crucial in critiquing a research hypothesis to determine whether it is a succinct statement of the relationship between two variables. Identify the variables in the following examples. Determine the independent variable and dependent variable in each of the following research hypotheses.

1. Regular provision of iron improves iron status of breast-fed infants without adverse effects (Zeigler, Nelson, & Jeter, 2009).

   a. Independent variable:

   b. Dependent variable:

2. Family-centered care (FCC) is a significant predictor of children's health-related quality of life (HRQL), independent of illness severity (Moore, Mah, & Trute, 2009).

   a. Independent variable:

   b. Dependent variable:

3. There is no difference between continuous nebulization of albuterol at 7.5 mg/hr (usual dose) and 15 mg/hr (high dose) in peak flow improvement up to 3 hours in the patients with acute bronchospasm (Stein & Levitt, 2003).

   a. Independent variable:

   b. Dependent variable:

4. People who report more frequent or more recent dental prophylaxes are more likely to have better glycemic control (Taylor et al., 2005).

   a. Independent variable:

   b. Dependent variable:

5. More supportive/less negative parenting is associated with lower resting blood pressure and heart rates in children (Bell & Belsky, 2008).

    a. Independent variable:

    b. Dependent variable:

Activity 5

Take each hypothesis from Activity 3 and label it with the appropriate abbreviation from the key provided. More than one abbreviation from the key may be used to describe each item.

Key: DH = Directional hypothesis
NDH = Nondirectional hypothesis
Hr = Research hypothesis
Ho = Statistical hypothesis

1. _____ Regular provision of iron improves iron status of breast-fed infants without adverse effects (Ziegler et al., 2009).

2. _____ Family-centered care (FCC) is a significant predictor of children's health-related quality of life (HRQL), independent of illness severity (Moore et al., 2009).

3. _____ There is no difference between continuous nebulization of albuterol at 7.5 mg/hr (usual dose) and 15 mg/hr (high dose) in peak flow improvement up to 3 hours in the patients with acute bronchospasm (Stein & Levitt, 2003).

4. _____ People who report more frequent or more recent dental prophylaxes are more likely to have better glycemic control (Taylor et al., 2005).

5. _____ More supportive/less negative parenting is associated with lower resting blood pressure and heart rates in children (Bell & Belsky, 2008).

Activity 6

Critique the following hypothesis.

African-American women with higher levels of depression will have higher blood pressure (BP) levels, more cardiovascular risk factors, greater stress, and lower social support (Artinian, Washington, Flack, et al., 2006).

1. Is the hypothesis clearly stated in a declarative form?

   Yes   No

2. Are the independent and dependent variables identified in the statement of the hypothesis?

   Yes   No

3. Are the variables measurable or potentially measurable?

   Yes   No

4. Is the hypothesis stated in such a way that it is testable?

   Yes   No

5. Is the hypothesis stated objectively without value-laden words?

    Yes   No

6. Is the direction of the relationship in the hypothesis clearly stated?

    Yes   No

7. Is each of the hypotheses specific to one relationship so that each hypothesis can be either supported or not supported?

    Yes   No

Activity 7

Clinical questions often arise from clinical situations. Using the PICO format for formulating clinical questions helps practicing nurses to identify the best available evidence on which to base clinical and health care decisions. In the following clinical questions, identify the four components of clinical questions.

1. In children presenting to the emergency department (ED) with acute long-bone fractures, is intranasal fentanyl equivalent to intravenous (IV) morphine for pain control? (Yost, 2007)

    P:

    I:

    C:

    O:

2. Is a group intervention for parents and children more effective than routine care for weight loss in obese school-age children? (Heale, 2008)

    P:

    I:

    C:

    O:

3. What are the experiences of men after laparoscopic radical prostatectomy (LRP)? (Mick, 2009)

    P:

    I:

    C:

    O:

POSTTEST

Refer to the article by Jones et al. (2007) in Appendix B of the text.

1. Highlight the research question.

2. Does the research question indicate a quantitative or qualitative research design?

3. Critique the research question by answering yes or no to the following questions. Does the research question

    a. Clearly identify the variable(s) under consideration?

    b. Specify the population being studied?

    c. Imply the possibility of empirical testing?

4. Put the research question into the PICO format for clinical questions.

5. List the variables being studied. Identify the independent variable(s) and dependent variable(s).

6. Is there a hypothesis stated by the researchers? If yes, highlight the hypothesis. Is the hypothesis directional or nondirectional?

REFERENCES

Artinian NT, Washington OGM, Flack JM, et al.: Depression, stress, and blood pressure in urban African-American women, *Prog Cardiovasc Nurs* 21(2):68-75, 2006.

Bell BG, Belsky J: Parenting and children's cardiovascular functioning, *Child Care Health Dev* 34(2):194-203, 2008.

Brown RA, Strong DR, Abrantes AM, et al.: Effects on substance use outcomes in adolescents receiving motivational interviewing for smoking cessation during psychiatric hospitalization, *Addictive Behaviors* 34(10):887-891, 2009.

Heale R: A group intervention for parents and children achieved greater weight loss in obese children than routine care, *Evidence Based Nursing* 11:43, 2008.

Jones EG, Renger R, Kang Y: Self-efficacy for health-related behaviors among deaf adults, *Res Nurs Health* 30:185-192, 2007.

Mick J: Men were surprised by the severity of symptoms they experienced after laparoscopic radical prostatectomy, *Evidence Based Nursing* 12:28, 2009.

Page RM, Lee C, Miao N: Self perception of body weight among high school students in Taipei, Taiwan, *Int J Adolesc Med Health* 17(2):123-136, 2005.

Rustøen T, Gaardsrud M, Leegaard M, Wahl AK: Nursing pain management: A qualitative interview study of patients with pain, hospitalized for cancer treatment, *Pain Manage Nurs* 10(1):48-55, 2009.

Shirrell D: Critical thinking as a predictor of success in an associate degree nursing program, *Teaching and Learning in Nursing* 3(4):131-136, 2008.

Stein J, Levitt MA: A randomized, controlled double-blind trial of usual-dose versus high-dose albuterol via continuous nebulization in patients with acute bronchospasm, *Ann Emerg Med* 10(1):31-36, 2003.

Taylor GW, Pritzel SJ, Manz MC, Borgnakke WS, Eber RM, Bouman PD (2005). Frequency of dental prophylaxis and glycemic control in type 2 diabetes. HYPERLINK "http://www.ingentaconnect.com/content/adha/jdh;jsessionid=7hnhm8si722gp.alice" \o "Journal of Dental Hygiene" *Journal of Dental Hygiene*, 79(4).

Winslow BW: Family caregivers' experiences with community services: A qualitative analysis, *Public Health Nurs* 20(5):341-348, 2003.

Yost J: Intranasal fentanyl and intravenous morphine did not differ for pain relief in children with closed long-bone fractures, *Evidence Based Nursing* 11:42, 2007.

Ziegler EE, Nelson SE, Jeter JM: Iron status of breastfed infants is improved equally by medicinal iron and iron-fortified cereal, *Am J Clin Nutr* 90(1):76-87, 2009.

Gathering and Appraising the Literature

INTRODUCTION

The term *review of the literature* or *literature review* refers to a key step in the research process for researchers, as well as for consumers of research. For researchers, the *literature review* refers to the section of a research study in which the researcher retrieves, critically appraises, and synthesizes previously existing knowledge. It is this *literature review* which is then used as the basis for the development of research questions and hypotheses by the researcher. Similarly, as consumers of research, nurses involved in evidence-based practice are also responsible for *reviewing the literature*. They systematically gather, critically appraise, and synthesize the best available evidence to determine the strength, quality, and consistency of the evidence to determine its applicability to practice. This chapter will help you learn more about how to critique the *literature review* performed by researchers and how to conduct a *literature review* as a consumer of research to address clinical questions.

LEARNING OUTCOMES

On completion of this chapter, the student should be able to do the following:

- Discuss the relationship of the literature review to nursing theory, research, education, and practice.
- Discuss the purposes of the literature review from the perspective of the research investigator and the research consumer.
- Discuss the use of the literature review for quantitative designs and qualitative methods.
- Discuss the purpose of reviewing the literature in development of evidence-based practice.
- Differentiate between primary and secondary sources.
- Compare the advantages and disadvantages of the most commonly used online databases and print database sources for conducting a literature review.
- Identify the characteristics of an effective electronic search of the literature.
- Critically read, appraise, and synthesize primary and secondary sources used for the development of a literature review.
- Apply critiquing criteria to the evaluation of literature reviews in selected research studies.

Activity 1

As a consumer of research, it is important to consider how a conceptual or theoretical framework guides the development of a study. In critically appraising a research study it is important to identify whether the researchers have used a conceptual or theoretical framework and how this framework has contributed to the development of the study's research questions and hypotheses. Refer to the study by Jones et al. (2007) (see Appendix B in the textbook) to answer the following questions.

1. Which, if any, theory is used by Jones et al. (2007) to guide their study?

2. What is the major concept being studied by Jones et al. (2007)?

3. Do the researchers provide a conceptual definition of this major concept, yes or no? If yes, what is the conceptual definition provided?

4. Do the researchers provide an operational definition of this major concept, yes or no? If yes, how is this concept being measured in this study?

Activity 2

Sometimes it is difficult to understand the distinction between primary and secondary sources of information. A comparison that is always helpful is if you are considering giving a client an injection for pain, whose report would you feel most comfortable evaluating—the report of a family member or nurse's aide (i.e., secondary source) or the report by the client (i.e., primary source)? As a consumer of nursing research, you will also need to evaluate the credibility of literature in part on whether they are generated from primary or secondary sources so that you know whether you are reading a first-hand report or someone else's interpretation of the material. Below is a selected list of references from the study by Jones et al. (2007) (Appendix B in the textbook). Next to each reference indicate whether it is a primary (*P*) or secondary (*S*) source. Sometimes it is helpful to retrieve the abstract or full text of the reference.

1. _____   Adler, N. E., & Newman, K. (2002). Socioeconomic disparities in health: Pathways and policies. *Health Affairs, 21*(2), 60-76.

2. _____   Allen, B., Meyers, N., Sullivan, J., & Sullivan, M. (2002). American Sign Language and end-of-life care: Research in the deaf community. *HEC Forum, 14*(3), 197-208.

3. _____   Bandura, A. (1986). *Social foundations of thought and action: A social cognitive theory.* Englewood Cliffs, NJ: Prentice-Hall.

4. _____   Baranowski, T., Perry, C. L., & Parcel, G. S. (2002). How individuals, environments, and health behavior interact. In K. Glanz, R. K. Rimer, & F. M. Lewis (Eds.). *Health behavior and health education: Theory, research, and practice* (pp. 165-184). San Francisco: Jossey-Bass.

5. _____ Barnett, S. (2002). Cross-cultural communication with patients who use American Sign Language. *Family Medicine, 34,* 376-382.

6. _____ Lang, H. G., McKee, B. G., & Conner, K. N. (1993). Characteristics of effective teachers: A descriptive study of perceptions of faculty and deaf college students. *American Annals of the Deaf, 138,* 252-259.

7. _____ Stebnicki, J. A. M., & Coeling, H. V. (1999). The culture of the deaf. *Journal of Transcultural Nursing, 10,* 350-357.

Activity 3

Typically a literature review consists of numerous journal articles. Whether the review of literature is being conducted by a researcher or consumer of research, attempts should be made to retrieve articles from refereed or peer-reviewed journals. Below is a selected list of references from the study by Jones et al. (2007) (Appendix B in the textbook). Next to each reference indicate whether it is a peer-reviewed journal (*PR*) or non peer-reviewed journal (*NPR*). Note: It may be helpful to look up the journal online.

1. _____ Barnett, S. (2002). Cross-cultural communication with patients who use American Sign Language. *Family Medicine, 34,* 376-382.

2. _____ Dolnick, E. (1993, September). Deafness as culture. *The Atlantic Monthly, 272*(3), 27-53.

3. _____ Hickey, M. L., Owen, S. V., & Froman, R. D. (1992). Instrument development: Cardiac diet and exercise self-efficacy. *Nursing Research, 41,* 247-351.

4. _____ Stebnicki, J. A. M., & Coeling, H. V. (1999). The culture of the deaf. *Journal of Transcultural Nursing, 10,* 350-357.

5. _____ Underwood, C. (2004). Maternity services are failing deaf women. *Journal of Family Health Care, 14*(2), 30-31.

Activity 4: Web-Based Activity

Although there remain books, journals, and additional literature that are only available in print versions located in libraries, the Internet has become a major source for researchers and consumers of research conducting reviews of the literature. Two of the most common internet sources are (1) online bibliographic and abstract databases and (2) online search engines. Conduct a search of CINAHL (the most relevant and frequently used source for nursing literature) and Google (an online search engine) using the following search terms: "postmenopausal women," "exercise," and "osteoporosis." Compare the literature retrieved.

1. How many items were retrieved from CINAHL?

2. How many items were retrieved from Google?

3. Which source retrieved the most relevant, peer-reviewed journal articles?

4. Which Internet source would be the best use of your time for gathering literature in a scholarly way?

Activity 5: Web-Based Activity

For the consumer of research, there are several barriers to conducting an exhaustive review of all of the available literature to answer a clinical question. Given this limitation, in the evidence-based model, nurses, as consumers of research, should be conducting a review of the literature to identify the best available evidence to answer a clinical question. Using your online libraries and bibliographic databases, conduct a search using the "5S" pyramid (see Figure 3-3 in your textbook) to identify the best available evidence to address the clinical question "Is diet or exercise more effective for long-term weight loss in adults?" Indicate the first three items retrieved under each of the categories of the "5S" pyramid. Note that you will be unable to search the highest level of the pyramid, computerized decision support systems, because few such systems are available at this time.

1. Summaries (clinical evidence)

    a. _____

    b. _____

    c. _____

2. Synopses (evidence-based nursing)

    a. _____

    b. _____

    c. _____

3. Syntheses (Cochrane Library or Cochrane Database of Systematic Reviews)

    a. _____

    b. _____

    c. _____

4. Studies (MEDLINE)

    a. _____

    b. _____

    c. _____

5. As a consumer of research, which "layer" of the "5S" pyramid provided you with the best available evidence to answer your clinical question?

Activity 6

The review of the literature is usually easy to find. In the abridged version of a research study it most frequently labeled *Review of Literature* or *Relevant Literature* or some other comparable term. It may also be separated into a literature review section and another section titled *Conceptual Framework* that presents material on the theoretical or conceptual framework. Critically appraising the literature review of research studies is a necessary step for both researchers and consumers of research. Refer to the study by Meneses et al. (2007) (see Appendix A in the textbook) to answer the following questions.

1. Are all relevant concepts and variables included in the review?

2. Does the search strategy include an appropriate and adequate number of databases and other resources to identify key published and unpublished research and theoretical sources?

3. Are both theoretical and research literature included?

4. Is there an appropriate theoretical/conceptual framework that guides the development of the research study?

5. Are primary sources mainly used?

6. What gaps or inconsistencies in knowledge does the literature review uncover?

7. Does the summary of each reviewed study reflect the essential components of the study design (e.g., type and size of sample, reliability and validity of instruments, consistency of data collection procedures, appropriate data analysis, identification of limitations)?

8. Does the synthesis summary follow a logical sequence that presents the overall strengths and weaknesses of the reviewed studies and arrive at a logical conclusion?

9. Is the literature review presented in an organized format that flows logically (e.g., chronologically, clustered by concept or variables), enhancing the reader's ability to evaluate the need for the particular research study or evidence-based practice project?

10. Does the literature review follow the proposed purpose of the research study or evidence-based practice project?

11. Does the literature review generate research questions or hypotheses or answer a clinical question?

Activity 7: Web-Based Activity

Retrieve and review the following articles:

Haynes RB: Of studies, summaries, synopses, summaries and systems: the "5S" evolution of information services for evidence-based healthcare decisions, *Evidence-Based Nursing* 10:6-7, 2007.
McKibbon KA, Marks S: Searching for the best evidence. Part 1: where to look, *Evidence-Based Nursing* 1:68-70, 1998.
McKibbon KA, Marks S: Searching for the best evidence. Part 2: searching CINAHL and Medline, *Evidence-Based Nursing* 1:105-107, 1998.

POSTTEST

Refer to the study by Horgas et al. (2008) (see Appendix C in the textbook) to answer the following questions.

1. Which, if any, theory is used by Horgas et al. (2007) to guide their study?

2. What is the major concept(s) being studied by Horgas et al. (2007)?

3. Do the researchers provide a conceptual definition of this major concept(s), yes or no? If yes, what is/are the conceptual definition(s) provided?

4. Do the researchers provide an operational definition(s) of the major concept(s), yes or no?

5. How is/are the major concept(s) being measured in this study?

6. Next to each of the references below from Meneses et al. (2008), indicate whether it is a primary (*P*) or secondary (*S*) source AND peer reviewed *(PR)* or not peer reviewed *(NPR)*.

   a. ____ ____   Bates, M. S., Edwards, W. T., & Anderson, K. O. (1993). Ethnocultural influences on variation in chronic pain perception. *Pain, 52,* 101-112.

   b. ____ ____   Edwards, C. L., Fillingim, R. B., & Keefe, F. (2001). Race, ethnicity, and pain. *Pain, 94,* 133-137.

   c. ____ ____   Bentler, P. M., & Bonett, D. G. (1980). Significance tests and goodness of fit in the analysis of covariance structures. *Psychological Bulletin, 88,* 588-606.

7. Are all relevant concepts and variables included in the review of the literature?

8. Does the search strategy include an appropriate and adequate number of databases and other resources to identify key published and unpublished research and theoretical sources?

9. Are both theoretical literature and research literature included?

10. Are primary sources mainly used?

11. What gaps or inconsistencies in knowledge does the literature review uncover?

12. Does the summary of each reviewed study reflect the essential components of the study design (e.g., type and size of sample, reliability and validity of instruments, consistency of data collection procedures, appropriate data analysis, identification of limitations)?

13. Does the synthesis summary follow a logical sequence that presents the overall strengths and weaknesses of the reviewed studies and arrive at a logical conclusion?

14. Is the literature review presented in an organized format that flows logically (e.g., chronologically, clustered by concept or variables), enhancing the reader's ability to evaluate the need for the particular research study or evidence-based practice project?

15. Does the literature review follow the proposed purpose of the research study or evidence-based practice project?

16. Does the literature review generate research questions or hypotheses or answer a clinical question?

REFERENCES

Haynes RB: Of studies, summaries, synopses, summaries and systems: The "5S" evolution of information services for evidence-based healthcare decisions, *Evidence-Based Nursing* 10:6-7, 2007.

Horgas AL, Yoon SL, Nichols AL, Marsiske M: The relationship between pain and functional disability in black and white older adults, *Res Nurs Health* 31:341-354, 2008.

Jones EG, Renger R, Kang Y: Self-efficacy for health-related behaviors among deaf adults, *Res Nurs Health* 30:185-192, 2007.

McKibbon KA, Marks S: Searching for the best evidence. Part 1: where to look, *Evidence-Based Nursing* 1:68-70, 1998.

McKibbon KA, Marks S: Searching for the best evidence. Part 2: searching CINAHL and Medline, *Evidence-Based Nursing* 1:105-107, 1998.

Meneses KD, McNees P, Loerzel V, et al.: Transition from treatment to survivorship: Effects of a psychoeducational intervention on quality of life in breast cancer survivors, *Oncol Nurs Forum* 34(5):1007-1016, 2007.

4

Introduction to Qualitative Research

INTRODUCTION

Using scientific methods is important for solving nursing problems. Although knowledge acquisition comes in a variety of ways, finding the optimal ways to answer nursing questions usually entails research. As nurses, we have a variety of assumptions and beliefs that influence the ways we see and interpret meanings about what is experienced. One might say that all research is about discovery, coming to know truth, and gaining knowledge. Historically, most have viewed science from its empirical perspectives and placed great value on scientific research, which focuses on *control, prediction, objectivity,* and *generalizability*, terms that will be discussed more thoroughly later. This perspective has the worldview that a single reality exists and aims to identify truth in objective and replicable ways. Empirical studies are essential for investigating particular variables, but are less helpful in understanding human responses and life experiences.

Whether researchers approach problems from quantitative or qualitative approaches, all are influenced by personal assumptions and beliefs. Some have vigorously argued about the worth of one scientific method over another. The quantitative approach to research has been viewed as successful in measuring and analyzing data, creating studies that can be replicated, and producing results that can be generalized to other populations. The quantitative method is usually referred to as *empirical analytical research*. Some have argued that qualitative methods are less rigorous than quantitative ones. Others say that because qualitative findings are not generalizable, this research method is less trustworthy. Despite the debates, many now agree that qualitative research is an important method for nursing research because some phenomena or observable events of interest to nursing are less easily measured using quantitative methods. Qualitative methods provide another means for discovering nursing knowledge and have become more respected forms of investigation over the last decade.

Qualitative research is a term often applied to naturalistic investigations, research that involves studying phenomena in places where they are occurring. Qualitative research approaches are based on a perceived perspective or holistic worldview that says there is not a single reality. Instead, reality is viewed as based on perceptions that differ from person to person and change over time; meaning can only be truly understood if it is associated with a specific situation or context. Qualitative research is about understanding phenomena and finding meaning through examining the pieces that make up the whole.

The most commonly used forms of qualitative nursing research methods are grounded theory, case study, ethnography, and phenomenology. Each method of investigation presents a unique approach to studying the phenomena of interest to nurses and the discipline.

Evidence-based practice has been primarily focused on findings that come from systematic reviews of the literature that use models focused on the effectiveness of interventions. As acceptance has grown for the use of evidence-based practice in nursing, old arguments about the place of qualitative research in this process have arisen. Since research designs such as case, descriptive, and evaluative studies continue to be valued less than empirical ones, it is important to understand the contributions made by qualitative research. Questions of interest to nursing that have not been previously or thoroughly studied are often best investigated using qualitative methods. When new perspectives are introduced to practice, the use of qualitative investigation may be the best way to gain early understandings that can later be studied using empirical measures. However, reviews of qualitative research about a given topic can also provide meaningful insight into practice issues that can be directly applied in clinical settings.

LEARNING OUTCOMES

On completion of this chapter, the student should be able to do the following:

- Describe the components of a qualitative research report.
- Differentiate between qualitative and quantitative research paradigms.
- Describe the beliefs generally held by qualitative researchers.
- Identify four ways qualitative findings can be used in evidence-based practice.

Activity 1

1. Before you go any further, and to be sure that you clearly understand the differences between quantitative and qualitative research, take some time to write a clear definition for each of the following terms:

   a. Quantitative research:

   b. Qualitative research:

2. Qualitative research occurs in naturalistic settings; list some potential settings where qualitative research may occur: _____

3. Qualitative research is _____ or _____ and uses _____ to describe a phenomenon.

Activity 2

In Chapter 4 of the textbook, the author provides an overview of qualitative research and introduces a variety of terms that have important implications for understanding qualitative research. Just as it is important to learn the vocabulary associated with quantitative research, this is also true with qualitative research. Take some time to define the following terms and be sure that you can differentiate them:

   a. Naturalistic settings:

   b. Context:

    c. Paradigm:

    d. Purposive sample:

    e. Inclusion and exclusion criteria:

    f. Data saturation:

    g. "Grand Tour" question:

Activity 3

Review Appendix D (Landreneau & Ward-Smith, 2007).

Find and summarize the following elements:

Elements of Landreneau & Ward-Smith, 2007

Element	Summary
Purpose	
Design	
Sample and setting	
Methods	
Inclusion criteria	

Activity 4

Think about your patient population and write a research question that would be best answered with a qualitative study for a phenomenon or experience that you are interested in.

Use Table 4-2 in the textbook to decide which mode of clinical application best relates to your research question.

Write research questions based on your topic to address the remaining clinical applications.

Activity 5: Web-Based Activity

Unless we have evidence assembled that demonstrates the way we are doing a particular procedure or continuing a specific protocol is less than adequate, most of us assume that because something is being done in nursing practice, it must be correct. Ideas about standards of practice, thoughts about best care, and concerns about quality are causing all practitioners to pay greater attention to questions about the evidence that does or does not support care decisions. While some nurses have embraced the concept of evidence-based care, others continue to be unclear about its implications and how to go about providing this form of care. Because most of the evidence-based studies are focused on quantitative studies often using clinical trials or intervention studies, less is known about the relationship between qualitative research and evidence-based care.

Take a few minutes to read the online paper titled "How Can We Argue for Evidence in Nursing?" at http://www.contemporarynurse.com/11.1/11-1p5.htm. This brief article suggests that nurses will make decisions about clinical care based on the best evidence available. However, many questions still exist about behavioral aspects of practice. For example, what is it like to be a young woman with type 1 diabetes who has suffered the complications of blindness and kidney failure, and spends 3 days a week associating with very ill elderly individuals on dialysis? Think for a few minutes about what that might be like. Then consider what evidence you would require to best deliver care to this individual if you were the nurse doing hemodialysis. What do you think might be known about the patient's experience or preference? What might not be known? Although much evidence may exist about the science of the care delivery, what is known that could be considered evidenced-based care in the way nursing care is delivered to meet the holistic needs of this particular patient? What kinds of resources and support might be needed that are different from other patients? Qualitative research enables one to investigate questions that are less easily answered through quantitative methods and can provide evidence that can directly affect care delivery.

POSTTEST

1. Identify whether each of the following beliefs reflects the quantitative or the qualitative research method:

   a. _____ Statistical explanation, prediction, and control

   b. _____ Neutral observer

   c. _____ Multiple realities exist

   d. _____ Objectivism valued

   e. _____ Active participant

   f. _____ Experimental

   g. _____ Dialogic

   h. _____ Time and place are important

   i. _____ One reality exists

   j. _____ Values add to understanding the phenomenon

2. Place the following components of a qualitative research report in order by numbering from 1 to 7 and provide a brief description of each.

   Data analysis:

   Sample:

   Review of the literature:

   Data collection:

Setting for recruitment and data collection:

Findings:

Study design:

REFERENCES

Landreneau KJ, Ward-Smith P: Perceptions of adult patients on hemodialysis concerning choice among renal replacement therapies, *Nephrol Nurs* 34(5):513-519, 525, 2007.

Street A: How can we argue for evidence in nursing? *Contemp Nurs* 11(1):5-8, 2001. Retrieved August 20, 2009, from www.contemporarynurse.com/archives/vol/11/issue/1/article/1496/how-can-we-argue-for-evidence-in-nursing.

Qualitative Approaches to Research

INTRODUCTION

Qualitative research continues to gain recognition as a sound method for investigating the complex human phenomena less easily explored using quantitative methods. Qualitative research methods provide ways to address both the science and art of nursing. Qualitative methods are especially well suited to address phenomena related to health and illness that are of interest to nurses and nursing practice. Nurse researchers and investigators from other disciplines are continuing to discover the value of findings obtained through qualitative studies. Nurses can be better prepared to critique the appropriateness of a research design and identify the usefulness of the study findings when the unique differences between quantitative and qualitative research approaches are understood.

Although there are many designs for qualitative research, five methods are most commonly used by nurses. These methods are phenomenology, grounded theory, ethnography, case study, and historical research. A newer methodology known as *community-based participatory research* that is gaining increased respect by nursing scientists who are investigating behavioral phenomena is also described in this chapter. Understanding and care are concepts related to behaviors that are important to nurses in the practice of clinical nursing care in a variety of settings across the lifespan. Each of these qualitative methods allows the researcher to approach the phenomena of interest from a different perspective. Each offers the investigator a different perspective and suggests findings that address different realms of human experience.

LEARNING OUTCOMES

On completion of this chapter, the student should be able to do the following:

- Identify the processes of phenomenological, grounded theory, ethnographic, and case study methods.
- Recognize appropriate use of historical methods.
- Recognize appropriate use of community-based participatory research methods.
- Discuss significant issues that arise in conducting qualitative research in relation to such topics as ethics, criteria for judging scientific rigor, and combination of research methods.
- Apply critiquing criteria to evaluate a report of qualitative research.

Activity 1

The reasons for selecting a qualitative design rather than a quantitative one are based on the type of research question asked and the study purpose. Recognizing the different characteristics of qualitative research from those of quantitative research enables the nurse to better understand the way the study was conducted, and interpret the research report findings. Clear understandings about qualitative research can also assist the nurse to better understand applications for the findings from these studies.

1. Complete the following statements related to qualitative research characteristics.

    a. Qualitative research combines the _____ and _____ natures of nursing to better understand the human experience.

    b. Qualitative research is used to study human experience and life context in _____ _____.

    c. Life context is the matrix of human-human-environment relationships that emerge over the course of _____ _____.

    d. Qualitative researchers study the _____ _____ of individuals as they carry on their usual activities of daily living, which might occur at home, work, or school.

    e. The number of participants or subjects in a qualitative study is usually _____ than the number in a quantitative study.

    f. Qualitative studies are intended to explore _____ _____ or _____ _____ in order to better understand the meanings ascribed by individuals living the experience.

    g. The choice to use either quantitative or qualitative methods is guided by the _____ _____.

    h. One research method is not better than another; it has to do with the _____ between one's worldview, the research question, and the research method.

2. Match the following definitions in Column A with the appropriate terms in Column B:

	Column A	Column B
a. _____	Information becomes repetitive	A. Theoretical sampling
b. _____	Select experiences to help the researcher test ideas and gather complete information about developing concepts	B. Emic
		C. Etic
		D. Data saturation
c. _____	Outsider's view	E. Secondary sources
d. _____	Identify personal biases about the phenomenon	
e. _____	Insider's view	F. Bracketed
f. _____	Symbolic categories	G. Case study method
g. _____	Individuals willing to teach investigator about the phenomenon	H. Grounded theory method
h. _____	In-depth description of the phenomenon	I. Domains
i. _____	Provide another perspective of the phenomenon	J. Key informants
j. _____	Inductive approach to develop theory about social processes	

3. Six qualitative research methods are discussed in the textbook in relation to five basic research elements. Use your textbook to compare research elements of each of the different types of qualitative methods. Briefly describe a key aspect of each element for the different qualitative methods. This activity will assist you to compare and contrast the similarities and differences in these methods.

    a. Element 1: Identifying the phenomenon

        1. Phenomenology

        2. Grounded theory method

        3. Ethnography

        4. Historical research

        5. Case study

        6. Community-based participatory research

    b. Element 2: Structuring the study

        1. Phenomenology

        2. Grounded theory method

        3. Ethnography

        4. Historical research

        5. Case study

        6. Community-based participatory research

    c. Element 3: Gathering the data

        1. Phenomenology

        2. Grounded theory method

      3.   Ethnography

      4.   Historical research

      5.   Case study

      6.   Community-based participatory research

  d. Element 4: Analyzing the data

      1.   Phenomenology

      2.   Grounded theory method

      3.   Ethnography

      4.   Historical research

      5.   Case study

      6.   Community-based participatory research

  e. Element 5: Describing the findings

      1.   Phenomenology

      2.   Grounded theory method

      3.   Ethnography

      4.   Historical research

      5.   Case study

      6.   Community-based participatory research

4. Take some time to think about an area of clinical practice that is of special interest to you. Consider questions or practice issues related to the clinical area. What kinds of problems do you think might be researched using qualitative perspectives? Make a list of two or three topics or problems that could be researched. Now identify the one that is of most interest to you. Based on the work you have just completed about the five elements of research methods, give some critical thought to the type of qualitative research that would be most appropriate for studying the identified problem. Once you have selected the type of qualitative research you would use, be prepared to explain the reasons for your choice.

Activity 2

The literature review usually provides the background and significance for understanding a research problem. All qualitative research methods do not include literature reviews, or if they do, they may tend to be much briefer than ones found in quantitative studies. The study in your text (Appendix D) titled "Perceptions of Adult Patients on Hemodialysis Concerning Choice Among Renal Replacement Therapies" by Landreneau and Ward-Smith (2007) includes a brief discussion about renal replacement therapy. Read the literature review at the beginning of this study report carefully, and then answer the following questions:

1. What is the main theme of the literature review?

2. How does this literature review introduce the reader to important problems associated with renal replacement therapies that might require research? What are the key points that the authors identify about the problem?

3. The authors say that this qualitative study followed a pilot study. What was it in the pilot study that drove the limitation to only hemodialysis patients in the larger study?

Activity 3

Read the methods section of the Landreneau and Ward-Smith (2007) report in Appendix D of your text and answer the following questions:

1. What research design was used to conduct this research study?

2. Describe the sample in this study.

3. What important procedures and methods were used to collect data in this study?

4. What methods were used during data analysis?

Activity 4

Qualitative research has many uses for nursing practice. After reading the Landreneau and Ward-Smith (2007) report in Appendix D of your text and considering the study findings, list some things learned and consider ways this research might be applicable to nursing practice.

Activity 5

Five qualitative methods of research are the phenomenological, grounded theory, ethnographic, case study, and historical methods. For each characteristic listed below, indicate which method of qualitative research it describes. Use the abbreviations from the key provided. Some characteristics may be described by more than one method.

Key:
    A = Phenomenological
    B = Grounded theory
    C = Ethnographic
    D = Historical
    E = Case study

a. _____   Uses primary and secondary sources

b. _____   Uses "emic" and "etic" views of subjects' worlds

c. _____   Research questions focus on basic social processes that shape behavior

d. _____   Central meanings arise from subjects' descriptions of lived experience

e. _____   Focuses on a dimension of day-to-day existence

f. _____   Uses theoretical sampling to analyze data

g. _____   Studies the peculiarities and commonalities of a specific case

h. _____   Discovers "domains" to analyze data

i. _____   Provides insight on the past and serves as a guide to the present and future

j. _____   Establishes fact, probability, or possibility

k. _____   States that individuals' history is a dimension of the present

l. _____   Attempts to discover underlying social forces that shape human behavior

m. _____   Attention is given to a single case

n. _____   Interviews "key informants"

o. _____   Presents data as a synthesized chronicle

p. _____   Focuses on describing cultural groups

q. _____   Uses constant comparative method during data analysis

r. _____   Researcher "brackets" personal bias or perspective

s. _____   Can include quantitative and/or qualitative data

t. _____   Subjects are currently experiencing a circumstance

u. _____   Collects remembered information from subjects

v. _____   Involves "field work"

w. _____   Describes events from the past

x. _____   May use photographs to describe current behavioral practices

y. _____   May not include exhaustive literature search

z. _____   Uses an inductive approach to understanding basic social processes

Activity 6

Critical thinking is an important aspect of all research. It is important to take some time to carefully consider all aspects of the research process before beginning. Based on the five methods of qualitative research described in the textbook, answer the following questions:

a. Select a qualitative method you found especially interesting and explain the two things you find appealing about this method.

b. Identify three subject areas for which this method might be helpful in developing nursing knowledge:

   (1)

   (2)

   (3)

c. Choose one of these subject areas and identify a research question to be studied.

d. Describe the data-collection methods you would use for this study.

e. Identify the characteristics of the study subjects, where you will locate them, how many subjects you might include, and why.

f. Briefly explain an important aspect of data analysis using this qualitative method.

g. Describe how you might use the knowledge gained from this study in nursing practice.

Activity 7: Web-Based Activity

Qualitative research is a way to develop knowledge about the complexity of the human health experience that occurs within a contextual setting during everyday life and over the lifespan. Chapter 5 in your textbook suggests that the use of qualitative research methods can provide evidence as findings are generated to (a) guide nursing practice, (b) contribute to development of instruments that can be used in quantitative research studies, and (c) develop nursing theory that can guide practice.

Go to *The Qualitative Report* at www.nova.edu/ssss/QR/web.html and see the large number of sources that can provide you additional understanding about qualitative research and assist you to understand better how the evidence produced by qualitative research is directly linked to nursing education, clinical practice, and research. Take some time to look over a few of these sites. You may want to select one that is related to the form of qualitative research that you have found especially intriguing. It is important that you begin to have some sense of the scope of work that is being done by nurses and others using qualitative methods. Although some continue to question the usefulness of these methods, the respect for and use of these means of scientific inquiry are continuing to grow.

After you have finished looking around, scroll down and select "Action Research on the Web." When the new page opens, choose "Action Research Electronic Reports." Select a report in an area of interest for you. Read through the article and then answer the following questions:

a. What was the research question?

b. What qualitative research method was used?

c. Reflect on how this study might become evidence for education or clinical practice.

POSTTEST

For questions 1 through 5, answer True (T) or False (F).

1. _____ Qualitative research focuses on the whole of human experience in naturalistic settings.

2. _____ *External criticism in historical research* refers to the authenticity of data sources.

3. _____ In qualitative research one would expect the number of subjects participating to be as large as those usually found in quantitative studies.

4. _____ The researcher is viewed as the major instrument for data collection.

5. _____ Qualitative studies strive to eliminate extraneous variables.

6. To what does the term *saturation* in qualitative research refer?
   a. Data repetition
   b. Subject exhaustion
   c. Researcher exhaustion
   d. Sample size

7. Data, in qualitative research, are often collected by which of the following procedures?
   a. Questionnaires sent out to subjects
   b. Observation of subjects in naturalistic settings
   c. Interviews
   d. All are correct

8. The qualitative method that uses an inductive approach using a systematic set of procedures to create a theory about basic social processes is known as which of the following?
   a. Phenomenology
   b. Grounded theory
   c. Ethnography
   d. Historical method

9. What is the qualitative method that attempts to construct the meaning of the lived experience of human phenomena?
   a. Phenomenology
   b. Grounded theory
   c. Ethnography
   d. Historical method
   e. Case study
   f. Community-based participatory research

10. What is the qualitative research method most appropriate for answering the question, "What changes in nursing practice occurred after the Vietnam War?"
    a. Phenomenology
    b. Grounded theory
    c. Ethnography
    d. Historical method
    e. Case study
    f. Community-based participatory research

11. What qualitative research method would be most appropriate for studying the impact of culture on the health behaviors of urban Hispanic youth?
    a. Phenomenology
    b. Grounded theory
    c. Ethnography
    d. Historical method
    e. Case study
    f. Community-based participatory research

12. What qualitative method would be most appropriate for studying a family's experience with cystic fibrosis?
    a. Phenomenology
    b. Grounded theory
    c. Ethnography
    d. Historical method
    e. Case study
    f. Community-based participatory research

13. What qualitative method would you use to study the spread of HIV/AIDS in an urban area?
    a. Phenomenology
    b. Grounded theory
    c. Ethnography
    d. Historical method
    e. Case study
    f Community-based participatory research

14. Which data analysis process is not used with grounded theory methodology?
    a. Bracketing
    b. Axial coding
    c. Theoretical sampling
    d. Open coding

REFERENCES

Landreneau KJ, Ward-Smith P: Perceptions of adult patients on hemodialysis concerning choice among renal replacement therapies, *Nephrol Nurs* 34(5):513-519, 525, 2007.

The Qualitative Report (July 3, 2009). Retrieved August 21, 2009, from www.nova.edu/ssss/QR/web.html.

6

Appraising Qualitative Research

INTRODUCTION

Qualitative research provides an opportunity to generate new knowledge about phenomena less easily studied with empirical or quantitative methods. Nurse researchers are increasingly using qualitative methods to explore holistic aspects less easily investigated with objective measures. In qualitative research, the data are less likely to involve numbers and most likely will include text derived from interviews, focus groups, observation, field notes, or other methods. The data tend to be mostly narrative or written words that require content rather than statistical analysis. The important contributions being made to nursing knowledge through qualitative studies make it important for nurses to possess skills that enable them to evaluate and critique qualitative research reports.

This chapter describes the criteria needed to evaluate and critique qualitative research reports. Qualitative researchers should provide the insider or emic view of the phenomenon being studied. Qualitative investigators often use a more conversational tone than what is found in quantitative research, and use quotations as a way to present the findings. Page limits in journals greatly constrain the ways investigators can present the richness of the data. Quotations selected must be chosen as exemplars that make the themes understandable to the reader. Published research reports, whether they are quantitative or qualitative, must be viewed by the reviewers as having scientific merit, demonstrate rigor in the research conducted, present new knowledge, and be of interest to the journal's readers. Qualitative research should offer evidence to enhance understanding or increase knowledge about a specific phenomenon; it may also have strong implications for evidence-based nursing practice.

LEARNING OUTCOMES

On completion of this chapter, the student should be able to do the following:

- Identify the influence of stylistic considerations on the presentation of a qualitative research report.
- Identify the criteria for critiquing a qualitative research report.
- Evaluate the strengths and weaknesses of a qualitative research report.
- Describe the applicability of the findings of a qualitative research report.
- Construct a critique of a qualitative research report.

Activity 1

The methods of presentation in qualitative research reports are different than those in quantitative studies. Nurses doing qualitative research reports are challenged to present the richness of the data within the restrictions of publication guidelines.

Review Appendix D, "Perceptions of Adult Patients on Hemodialysis Concerning Choice Among Renal Replacement Therapies" by Landreneau and Ward-Smith (2007), to identify the ways the researchers stylistically presented the rich data. In the finding section titled "Theme One: Knowledge," the researchers describe several aspects of this process and give examples from the data to describe what is implied. Carefully read this section and identify the descriptive examples or quotations that summarize the key points.

Activity 2

The findings of qualitative studies describe or explain a phenomenon within a specific context. The findings are not usually intended to be generalizable to other groups, which means that people who want to apply the findings to others have the responsibility to validate whether the findings are applicable in a different setting and with other people or populations.

Review the sections titled "Findings," "Discussion," and "Conclusions" from "Perceptions of Adult Patients on Hemodialysis Concerning Choice Among Renal Replacement Therapies" by Landreneau and Ward-Smith (2007). After you have reviewed the article, answer the following questions:

1. What does the study conclude about perceptions of choice in renal replacement?

2. What does the study say about generalizability of this study?

3. What do the authors suggest about patients' knowledge?

4 List three potential studies to follow up on the findings from this research.

Activity 3

Critiquing qualitative research enables the nurse to make sense out of the research report, build on the body of knowledge about human phenomena, and consider how knowledge might be applicable to nursing. Learning and applying a critiquing process is the first step in this process.

1. Review Critiquing Criteria Box on page 129 in the text and match the activity in Column A with the qualitative research process in Column B. Some steps are used more than once.

Column A

a. _____ The purpose of the study is clearly stated.

b. _____ Audiotaped interviews were used to collect phenomenological data.

c. _____ Do the participants recognize the experience as their own?

d. _____ Purposive sampling was used.

e. _____ Data are clearly reported in the research report.

f. _____ The researcher has remained true to the findings.

g. _____ Recommendations for future research are made.

h. _____ The phenomenon of interest is clearly identified.

i. _____ Participant observation was done in an ethnography.

Column B

A. Subject selection
B. Study method
C. Researcher perspective
D. Data analysis
E. Application of findings
F. Findings description
G. Study design

2. Define the following terms:

a. Credibility:

b. Auditability:

c. Fittingness:

d. Saturation:

e. Trustworthiness:

Activity 4: Web-Based Activity

The Internet can be a valuable tool in gaining insight into qualitative research topics. Searching the term *qualitative research* can be a way to gain additional understanding about many aspects of this research approach. However, it is essential to identify a few quality starting points for your investigation. The University of Alberta's International Institute for Qualitative Methodology at www.ualberta.ca/~iiqm/ is an excellent place to locate information about conferences, journals, training, and international research. Start from the University of Alberta site and follow the link to the *International Journal of Qualitative Methods*. Search for the term *experience* and note the variety of research methodologies used to explore this concept. Another good site is Judy Norris's "QualPage" at www.qualitativeresearch.uga.edu/QualPage/, a valuable resource for learning more about the various methods of qualitative research.

You may want to spend some time reviewing these websites to learn more about the state of qualitative research methods. Your instructor may want to assign some particular activities from these websites to assist you in learning about qualitative research.

POSTTEST

For questions 1 through 6, answer True (T) or False (F).

1. _____ Qualitative research findings are generalizable to other groups.

2. _____ Findings from qualitative research designs are viewed as less credible by nurse researchers than those gained from quantitative studies.

3. _____ Auditability is an important aspect of evaluating a qualitative research report.

4. _____ The style of a qualitative research report differs from that of a quantitative research report.

5. _____ Some journal publication guidelines may impede the qualitative researcher's ability to convey the richness of the data.

6. _____ Journal reviewer's guidelines usually allow for the extra pages that qualitative researchers might need to provide the detail of their rich data.

7. _____ means that others should be able to identify the thinking, decisions, and methods used by the researchers when they conducted the research study.

8. _____ means that the study findings fit well outside the study situation.

9. _____ means that the research informants can identify the reported findings as their own experience.

10. _____ are the terms usually applied to qualitative research to judge the validity and reliability of qualitative data.

REFERENCES

Landreneau KJ, Ward-Smith P: Perceptions of adult patients on hemodialysis concerning choice among renal replacement therapies, *Nephrol Nurs* 34(5):513-519, 525, 2007.

Norris J: QualPage: Resources for Qualitative Research. Retrieved August 21, 2009, from www.qualitativeresearch.uga.edu/QualPage/.

University of Alberta: International Institute for Qualitative Methodology. Retrieved August 21, 2009, from www.ualberta.ca/~iiqm/.

7

Introduction to Quantitative Research

INTRODUCTION

The term *research design* is used to describe the overall plan of a particular study. The design is the researcher's plan for answering specific research questions in the most accurate and efficient way possible. In quantitative research, the plan outlines how the hypotheses will be tested. The design ties together the present research problem, the knowledge of the past, and the implications for the future. Thus the choice of a design reflects the researcher's experience, expertise, knowledge, and biases.

LEARNING OUTCOMES

On completion of this chapter, the student should be able to do the following:

- Define *research design.*
- Identify the purpose of research design.
- Define *control* as it affects research design.
- Compare and contrast the elements that affect control.
- Begin to evaluate what degree of control should be exercised in research design.
- Define *internal validity.*
- Identify the threats to internal validity.
- Define *external validity.*
- Identify the conditions that affect external validity.
- Identify the links between the study design and evidence-based practice.
- Evaluate research design using critiquing questions.

Activity 1

Match the definition of the terms in Column A with the research design terms in Column B. Each term is used no more than once, and not all terms will be used. Check the glossary for help with terms.

	Column A		Column B
1. _____	A sample of subjects similar to one another	a.	External validity
2. _____	The subject's responses to being studied	b.	Internal validity
		c.	Accuracy
3. _____	Methods to keep the study conditions constant during the study	d.	Research design
		e.	Control
4. _____	Consideration of whether the study is possible and practical to conduct	f.	Random sampling
		g.	Feasibility
		h.	Homogenous sampling
5. _____	The vehicle for hypothesis testing or answering research questions	i.	Objectivity
		j.	Reactivity
6. _____	Process to ensure every subject has an equal chance of being selected		
7. _____	Degree to which a research study is consistent within itself		
8. _____	Degree to which the study results can be applied to the larger population		
9. _____	All parts of a study follow logically from the problem statement		

Activity 2

For each of the following situations, identify the type of threat to internal validity from the list below. Then explain the reason this is a problem, and suggest how this problem can be corrected.

History	Mortality
Instrumentation	Selection bias
Maturation	Testing

1. The researcher tested the effectiveness of a new method of teaching drug dosage and solution calculations to nursing students using a standardized calculation examination at the beginning, midpoint, and end of a 2-week course.

2. In a study of the results of a hypertension teaching program conducted at a senior center, the blood pressures taken by volunteers using their personal equipment were compared before and after the program.

3. A major increase in cigarette taxes occurs during a 1-year follow-up study of the impact of a smoking cessation program.

4. The smoking cessation rates of an experimental group consisting of volunteers for a smoking cessation program were compared with the results of a control group of people who wanted to quit on their own without a special program.

5. Thirty percent of the subjects dropped out of an experimental study of the effect of a job-training program on employment for homeless women. Over 90% of the dropouts were single homeless women with at least two preschool children, whereas the majority of subjects successfully completing the program had no preschool children.

6. Nurses on a maternity unit want to study the effect of a new hospital-based teaching program on mothers' confidence in caring for their newborn infants. A survey is mailed to participants by the researchers 1 month after discharge.

Activity 3

The term *research design* is an all-encompassing term for the overall plan to answer the research questions, including the method and specific plans to control other factors that could influence the results of the study. To become acquainted with the major elements in the design of a study, read the Jones, Renger, and Kang (2007) article (Appendix B in the text) and answer the following questions:

a. What was the setting for the study?

b. Who were the subjects?

c. How was the sample selected?

d. What were the exclusion criteria?

e. Was this a homogenous sample?

  f. What instruments were used, what type of data was collected, and how was constancy maintained between groups?

  g. Which group served as the control group?

Activity 4

Use the critiquing criteria in Chapter 7 to critique the research design of the Meneses et al. study (2007) (see Appendix A). Explain your answers.

  1. Is the design appropriate?

  2. Is the control consistent with the research design?

  3. Think about the feasibility of this study. What are some of the feasibility challenges for this study?

  4. Does the design logically flow from problem, framework, literature review, and hypothesis?

  5. What are the threats to internal validity and how did the investigators control for each?

  6. What are the threats to external validity and how did the investigators control for each?

Activity 5: Web-Based Activity

Assume you are thinking about submitting a proposal to the National Institute of Nursing Research (NINR). You are a multitalented researcher and are equally qualified to conduct either qualitative or quantitative research. You are curious about the number of grants awarded that would be considered quantitative or qualitative. Start at the NINR website and describe how you could use this site to get a sense of the qualitative/quantitative ratio.

  Go to www.ninr.nih.gov/. Click on each of the following in order:

- "Research and Funding"
- "Funded NINR Grants/Collaborative Activities"
- Look for the most recent year

Review the studies that appear. Do these titles give you enough information to determine if the awarded grant was qualitative or quantitative in nature? Read through the first 10 citations and label them as either qualitative or quantitative.

Note: URLs for websites may change. If you receive an error message at the URL listed above, go to your favorite search engine and type in "National Institute of Nursing Research"; this should lead you to the desired site.

An excellent source of information about both quantitative and qualitative studies can be your own university library. Go to your campus home page and type in "library," then type in "research" or "nursing research." This can be an excellent source for full-text journals; however, they are usually password-protected, so you will need to obtain a password from your library to access them.

Activity 6: Evidence-Based Practice Activity

Review Figure 1-1, "Levels of evidence: evidence hierarchy for rating levels of evidence, associated with a study's design," from your text below. For each level of evidence, match the level of evidence in the left column to the description in the right column. For each level, indicate whether the evidence is (A) expert opinion, (B) qualitative, (C) quantitative, (D) combination of qualitative and quantitative, or (E) anecdotal.

Level of Evidence	Answers		Description
1. Level I:			a. Single descriptive or qualitative study
2. Level II:			b. A well-designed RCT
3. Level III:			c. Meta-analysis of RCTs
4. Level IV:			d. Systematic review of qualitative studies
5. Level V:			e. Opinion of authorities; reports of expert committees
6. Level VI:			f. Quasi-experimental study
7. Level VII:			g. Single nonexperimental study

POSTTEST

1. Review the Meneses et al. study (2007) (see Appendix A). Briefly assess the major components of the research design.

    a. Use your own words to state the purpose of the study.

    b. What is the setting for the study?

    c. Who are the subjects?

    d. How is the sample selected?

    e. What is the research treatment?

    f. How do the researchers attempt to control elements affecting the results of the study?

2. Fill in the blanks by selecting from the following list of terms. Not all terms will be used.

Constancy   Mortality
Control   Internal validity
Feasibility   External validity
Selection bias   Accuracy
Reliability   History
Maturation

a. _____ is used to hold steady the conditions of the study.

b. _____ is used to describe that all aspects of a study logically follow from the problem statement.

c. The believability between this study and the world at large is known as _____.

d. The developmental, biological, or psychological processes known as _____ operate within a person over time and may influence the results of a study.

e. Time, subject availability, equipment, money, experience, and ethics are factors influencing the _____ of a study.

f. Selection bias, mortality, maturation, instrumentation, testing, and history influence the _____ of a study.

g. Voluntary (rather than random) assignment to an experimental or control condition creates a situation known as _____.

REFERENCES

Jones EG, Renger R, Kang Y: Self-efficacy for health-related behaviors among deaf adults, *Res Nurs Health* 30:185-192, 2007.

Meneses DK, McNees P, Loerzel W, et al.: Transition from treatment to survivorship: Effects of a psychoeducational intervention on quality of life in breast cancer survivors, *Oncol Nurs Forum* 34:1007-1016, 2007.

National Institute of Nursing Research: Retrieved August 21, 2009, from http://ninr.nih.gov/.

8

Experimental and Quasi-Experimental Designs

INTRODUCTION

This chapter contains exercises for two categories of design: experimental and quasi-experimental designs. These types of designs allow researchers to test the effects of nursing actions and make statements about cause-and-effect relationships. Therefore they can be very helpful in testing solutions to nursing practice problems. However, a researcher chooses the design that allows a given situation or problem to be studied in the most accurate and effective way possible. Thus not all problems are amenable to immediate study by these two types of designs. Rather, the choice of design is dependent on the development of knowledge relevant to the problem, plus the researcher's knowledge, experience, expertise, preferences, and resources.

LEARNING OUTCOMES

On completion of this chapter, the student should be able to do the following:

- Describe the purpose of experimental and quasi-experimental research.
- Describe the characteristics of experimental and quasi-experimental studies.
- Distinguish the differences between experimental and quasi-experimental designs.
- List the strengths and weaknesses of experimental and quasi-experimental designs.
- Identify the types of experimental and quasi-experimental designs.
- List the criteria necessary for inferring cause-and-effect relationships.
- Identify potential validity issues associated with experimental and quasi-experimental designs.
- Critically evaluate the findings of experimental and quasi-experimental studies.
- Identify the contribution of experimental and quasi-experimental designs to evidence-based practice.

Activity 1

Fill in the blank for each of the following descriptions with a term selected from the list of types of experimental and quasi-experimental designs. Each term is used only once and not all terms may be used. Consult the glossary for assistance with definition of terms.

After-only experiment   Nonequivalent control group
After-only nonequivalent control group   Solomon four-group
True experimental   Time series
One-group design

1. _____ designs are particularly suitable for testing cause-and-effect relationships because they help eliminate potential alternative explanations (threats to validity) for the findings.

2. The type of design that has two groups identical to the true experimental design plus an experimental after-group and a control after-group is known as a(n) _____ _____ design.

3. A research approach used when only one group is available to study for trends over a longer period of time is called a(n) _____ design.

4. The _____ design is also known as the posttest-only control group design in which neither the experimental group nor the control group is pretested.

5. If a researcher wants to compare results obtained from an experimental group with a control group, but was unable to conduct pretests or to randomly assign subjects to groups, the study would be known as a(n) _____ design.

6. The _____ design includes three properties: randomization, control, and manipulation.

7. When subjects are unable to be randomly assigned into experimental and control groups but are able to be pretested and posttested, the design is known as a(n) _____ _____ design.

Activity 2

Review the study by Jones, Renger, and Kang (2007) titled "Self-Efficacy for Health-Related Behaviors Among Deaf Adults" (see Appendix B) and then answer the following questions.

1. What is the name of the design used in this study?

2. Explain this type of design.

3. What are the events that could be labeled antecedent variables and intervening variables in the study that could have affected internal validity?

    a. Which events would be labeled an antecedent variable?

    b. Which would be labeled an intervening variable?

4. List the implications of this study for nursing practice.

Activity 3

The education department in a large hospital wants to test a program to educate and change nurse's attitudes regarding pain management. They have a questionnaire that measures nurses' knowledge and attitudes about pain. Your responsibility is to design a study to examine the outcome of this intervention program.

1. You decide to use a Solomon four-group design. Complete the chart below with an X to indicate which of the four groups receive the pretest and posttest pain questionnaire and which receive the experimental teaching program.

	Pretest	Teaching	Posttest
Group A	_____	_____	_____
Group B	_____	_____	_____
Group C	_____	_____	_____
Group D	_____	_____	_____

2. How would you assign nurses to each of the four groups?

3. What would you use as a pretest for the groups receiving the pretest?

4. What is the experimental treatment?

5. What is the outcome measure for each group?

6. Based on your reading, for what types of issues is this design particularly effective?

7. What is the major advantage for this type of design?

8. What is a disadvantage for this type of design?

Activity 4

For each of the following descriptions of experimental or quasi-experimental studies, identify the type of design used in the study and the advantages and disadvantages of this design.

1. The purpose of this study was to test the effectiveness of the Deaf Heart Health Intervention (DHHI) in increasing self-efficacy for health-related behaviors among deaf adults. Eighty-four participants completed the Self-Rated Abilities Scale for Health Practices (SRAHP) in sign language, 32 participants completed the DHHI, and 52 were in the comparison group (Jones, Renger, & Kang, 2007).

   a. Based on the short description above, what types of design could have been used? Review the study in Appendix B and explain why the authors chose the type of design they used. (Think it through; this design is a combination of two of the designs addressed in the text.)

   b. What are the advantages of this design?

   c. What are the disadvantages of this design?

2. The purpose of this study was to examine the effectiveness of a psychoeducational intervention on quality of life in breast cancer survivors in posttreatment survivorship. Sample consisted of 256 breast cancer survivors who were randomly assigned to the experimental or wait-control group (Meneses et al., 2007).

   a. What type of design was used?

   b. What is the benefit of using a "wait-control" or "attention-control" group?

   c. What was the dependent variable?

   d. What was the independent variable?

Activity 5

1. You may be questioning why anyone would use a quasi-experimental design if an experimental design has the advantage of being so much stronger in detecting cause-and-effect relationships and enabling the researcher to generalize the results to a wider population. In what instances might it be advantageous to use a quasi-experimental design?

2. What must the researcher do in order to generalize the findings from a quasi-experimental research study?

3. What must a clinician do before application of research findings into practice?

Activity 6: Web-Based Activity

In this activity, you are looking for experimental nursing research studies.

1. Use your library access to enter PubMed or go to www.ncbi.nlm.nih.gov/pubmed/ and type in "experimental studies nursing." How many articles were found?

2. Look at the first 10 articles. Are they actual experimental studies? If not, what are they?

3. Now click on the "Limits" tab near the top. In the "Type of article" choose the option "Randomized Control Trial." Click on "Go." How many articles were found with this limit set?

4. Now click on the "Limits" tab near the top. In the "Subsets" menu choose the option "nursing journals." Click on "Go." How many articles were found with this limit set?

Activity 7: Evidence-Based Practice Activity

When using evidence-based practice strategies, the first step is to decide which level of evidence a research article provides. Review Figure 1-1, Levels of evidence: Evidence hierarchy for rating levels of evidence, associated with a study's design below from your textbook.

1. Review the Jones, Renger, and Kang (2007) article (see Appendix B). Then select the appropriate level of evidence category for this study, Level I through Level VII.

2. Review the Meneses et al. (2007) article (see Appendix A). Then select the appropriate level of evidence category for this study.

POSTTEST

1. Identify whether the following studies are (E) experimental or (Q) quasi-experimental designs.

   a. _____ Fifty teen mothers are randomly assigned into an experimental parenting support group and a regular support group. Before the program and at the end of the 3-month program, mother-child interaction patterns are compared between the two groups.

   b. _____ Patients on two separate units are given a patient satisfaction with care questionnaire to complete at the end of their first hospital day and on the day of discharge. The patients on one unit receive care directed by a nurse case manager, and the patients on the other unit receive care from the usual rotation of nurses. Patient satisfaction scores are compared.

   c. _____ Students are randomly assigned to two groups. One group receives an experimental independent study program and the other receives the usual classroom instruction. Both groups receive the same posttest to evaluate learning.

   d. _____ A study was conducted to compare the effectiveness of a music relaxation program with silent relaxation on lowering blood pressure ratings. Subjects were randomly assigned into groups and blood pressures were measured before, during, and immediately after the relaxation exercises.

   e. _____ Reading and language development skills were compared between a group of children with chronic otitis media and a group of children without a history of ear problems.

2. Identify the type of experimental or quasi-experimental design for each of the following examples. Use the numbers from the key provided.

   Key: 1 = After-only
   2 = After-only nonequivalent control group
   3 = True experiment
   4 = Nonequivalent control group
   5 = Time series
   6 = Solomon four-group

   a. _____ Nurses are randomly assigned to a new self-study program or the usual ECG teaching program. Knowledge of ECGs is tested before and after the program for both groups.

   b. _____ Babies who tested positive on toxicology screening at birth are randomly assigned into groups to either receive routine care or to receive a special public health nurse intervention program. Health outcomes are tested and compared at 6 months.

   c. _____ A school nurse clinic is set up at one school. Health care outcomes are measured at the end of a year from that school and compared with health outcomes at a comparable school that does not have a clinic.

   d. _____ Diabetic patients were randomly assigned to either one of two control groups receiving routine home health care or to one of two groups with a new diabetic teaching program. Patients in one of the control groups and in one of the teaching groups took a test of diabetic knowledge as soon as they were assigned to a group. Patients in the other two groups were not pretested. All patients completed a posttest at the conclusion of the 3-week program.

e. _____ A new peer AIDS prevention program was implemented in one high school. A second high school without the program served as a control group. An AIDS knowledge test was administered at both schools before and after the program was completed.

f. _____ Trends in patient falls were summarized each week 1 year before and for the first year after implementation of a new hospital-based quality assurance program.

REFERENCES

Jones EG, Renger R, Kang Y: Self-efficacy for health-related behaviors among deaf adults, *Res Nurs Health* 30:185-192, 2007.

Meneses DK, McNees P, Loerzel W, et al.: Transition from treatment to survivorship: Effects of a psychoeducational intervention on quality of life in breast cancer survivors, *Oncol Nurs Forum* 34:1007-1016, 2007.

Nonexperimental Designs

INTRODUCTION

Nonexperimental designs can provide extensive amounts of data that can help fill in the gaps found in nursing research. These designs help us clarify, see the real world, and assess relationships between variables, and they can provide clues to direct future, more controlled research. In this way, experimental, quasi-experimental, and nonexperimental designs complement each other. Each provides necessary components of our knowledge base. Nonexperimental designs allow us to discover some of the territory of nursing knowledge before trying to rearrange parts of it. It can be the base on which knowledge is built and further refined with quasi-experimental and experimental research.

LEARNING OUTCOMES

On completion of this chapter, the student should be able to do the following:

- Describe the overall purpose of nonexperimental designs.
- Describe the characteristics of survey, relationship, and difference designs.
- Define the differences among survey, relationship, and difference designs. List the advantages and disadvantages of surveys and each type of relationship and difference designs.
- Identify methodological and secondary analysis methods of research.
- Identify the purposes of methodological and secondary analysis methods of research.
- Describe the purposes of a systematic review, meta-analysis, integrative review, and clinical practice guidelines.
- Define the differences among a systematic review, meta-analysis, integrative review, and clinical practice guidelines.
- Discuss relational inferences versus causal inferences as they relate to nonexperimental designs.
- Identify the critical appraisal criteria used to critique nonexperimental research designs.
- Apply the critiquing criteria to the evaluation of nonexperimental research designs as they appear in research reports.
- Apply the critiquing criteria to the evaluation of systematic reviews and clinical practice guidelines.
- Evaluate the strength and quality of evidence by nonexperimental designs.
- Evaluate the strength and quality of evidence provided by systematic reviews, meta-analysis, integrative reviews, and clinical practice guidelines.

Activity 1

Determine an answer for each of the following items. Once you have an answer, study the diagram to find each answer. The words will always be in a straight line. They may be read up or down, left to right, right to left, or diagonally. When you find one of the words, draw a circle around it. Any single letter may be used in more than one word, but when the puzzle is finished, not all words will be used. There are no spaces or hyphens between the words in the puzzle; thus if it is a multiword answer, link the letters together as if it is all one word. Some of the terms will be used more than once to fill in the blanks in the statements below.

Experimental Design Puzzle

```
L  O  N  G  I  T  U  D  I  N  A  L  D  M  E
C  I  S  P  U  E  Q  W  H  X  O  I  Y  H  X
C  R  F  L  G  Y  Q  E  R  C  X  E  C  G  P
U  W  O  L  Z  S  B  Q  F  H  V  O  H  H  O
N  T  L  S  C  I  S  Z  A  R  R  O  I  U  S
L  G  T  R  S  D  L  D  U  R  Z  L  D  O  T
U  E  I  O  I  S  Q  S  E  D  L  V  W  O  F
I  U  W  S  J  J  E  L  O  S  Y  U  H  I  A
G  T  D  K  X  O  A  C  I  E  M  D  I  I  C
Q  W  R  E  E  T  O  K  T  T  E  S  T  A  T
A  S  A  M  I  K  E  N  B  I  B  H  U  L  O
D  U  O  O  K  L  H  N  P  H  O  B  Z  V  F
M  C  N  G  U  L  U  E  O  L  Y  N  R  K  C
K  A  M  F  G  U  P  Q  S  B  Z  L  A  H  T
L  W  J  F  V  N  E  W  J  S  W  L  E  L  V
```

1. This type is better known for the breadth than the depth of data collected. _____

2. A major disadvantage is the length of time needed for data collection. _____

3. The main question is whether or not variables co-vary. _____

4. These words mean *after the fact.* _____

5. This eliminates the confounding variable of maturation. _____

6. This quantifies the magnitude and direction of a relationship. _____

7. Collects data from the same group at several points in time. _____

8. Can be surprisingly accurate if the sample is representative. _____

9. Uses data from one point in time. _____

10. This is based on two or more naturally occurring groups with different conditions of the presumed independent variable. _____

Activity 2

Listed below are a series of advantages and disadvantages for various types of nonexperimental designs. For each type of design, pick at least one advantage (A) and one disadvantage (D) from the list that accurately describes a quality of the design. Then insert the A or D and the appropriate number in the list below.

	Advantages	**Disadvantages**
Correlation studies	_____	_____
Cross-sectional	_____	_____
Ex post facto	_____	_____
Longitudinal	_____	_____
Prospective	_____	_____
Retrospective	_____	_____
Survey	_____	_____

Advantages

A1 A great deal of information can be economically obtained from a large population.

A2 Ability to assess changes in the variables of interest over time.

A3 Explores relationship between variables that are inherently not manipulable.

A4 Offers a higher level of control than a correlational study.

A5 They facilitate intelligent decision making, using objective criteria to guide the process.

A6 Each subject is followed separately and serves as his or her own control.

A7 Stronger than retrospective studies because of the degree of control on extraneous variables.

A8 Less time-consuming, less expensive, and thus more manageable for the researcher.

Disadvantages

D1 The inability to draw a causal linkage between two variables.

D2 An alternative hypothesis could be the reason for the relationships.

D3 The researcher is unable to manipulate the variables of interest.

D4 The researcher is unable to determine a causal relationship between variables because of lack of manipulation, control, and randomization.

D5 The information obtained tends to be superficial.

D6 The researcher must know sampling techniques, questionnaire construction, interviewing, and data analysis.

D7 No randomization in sampling because studying preexisting groups.

D8 Internal validity threats such as testing and mortality are present.

D9 Subject loss to follow-up and attrition may lead to unintended sample bias that affects external validity and generalizability of findings.

Activity 3

All of the following are descriptions of nonexperimental studies. For each example, determine the type of design utilized from the list provided. Not all designs are used as examples, and some will be used more than once.

C	Correlation studies
CS	Cross-sectional
E	Ex post facto
L	Longitudinal
M	Methodological
MA	Meta-analysis
P	Prospective
R	Retrospective
SC	Survey comparative
SD	Survey descriptive
SE	Survey exploratory

Remember, some studies use more than one type of nonexperimental design.

1. A public health education nurse working with a senior center surveyed all residents to determine their priorities for health education classes and events.

   Type of design:

2. A study of children ages 2 to 18 with diabetes collected data every year. Information collected included health surveys, $HgbA_{1c}$ levels, 24-hour diet recall, and measurements of height and weight. Children were assessed yearly and were included in the study up to age 18; data were collected for 10 consecutive years.

   Type of design:

3. In a study of 200 low-income seniors, approximately half were Caucasian and half were African American. Explored the relationship among hypertension, depression, self-esteem, and health-seeking behaviors. The data were collected on one occasion.

   Type of design:

4. A study examined the relationship of maternal dietary choices and infant birth weight. Medical records of 1,000 postpartum women were examined to determine dietary choices and the relationship of a vegetarian or vegan diet to infant birth weight.

   Type of design:

5. An exploration of the relationship between hypertension and social interaction in elderly adults living in isolated rural areas.

   Type of design:

6. Forty-seven items were initially developed for the Haber and Wood Student Assessment Tool (HWSAT) after a thorough examination of the literature. These items were reviewed for relevance to the domain of content by a panel of eight experts using content validation.

   Type of design:

7. The purpose of this study is to examine the effect of simulation in nursing education and pass rates on board examinations. The LoBiondo-Wood Model of concept development was used in this study. An electronic search of the literature in several databases (CINAHL, MEDLINE, PubMed, Scopus) was conducted to find studies of the effectiveness of simulation on board exam pass rates in the nursing literature. The 23 quantitative studies meeting critiquing criteria were included in this study, which used statistical analysis to evaluate the effect of simulation on board pass rates.

   Type of design:

Activity 4

Use the critiquing criteria from the chapter to analyze the article from Rice and Stead (2008) (see Appendix E). In this article, the objective was to determine the effectiveness of nursing-delivered smoking cessation interventions by extracting data from RCTs. The sample consisted of 42 studies of smoking cessation interventions delivered by nurses with follow-up for at least 6 months.

1. Type of design:

2. Were the inclusion and exclusion criteria for studies included in the analysis? If so, what were they?

3. Where would you find the search terms and dates included in the database searches? What were the search terms?

4. Are the studies assessed using a quality index or criteria? Describe the criteria if used.

Activity 5

Review the Critical Thinking Decision Path: Nonexperimental Design Choice found in the textbook. If you wanted to test a relationship between two variables in the past such as the incidence of reported back injuries of nurses working in newborn nursery compared with those nurses working in long-term care, which design would you use?

Activity 6: Web-Based Activity

This activity will assist you in finding nursing research survey instruments if you are considering gathering data for a nonexperimental survey study. Use two search engines (Google, Google Scholar) and one website (PubMed) to find instruments, and then compare the three sources to determine which is the most helpful to you.

1. First, go to the National Library of Medicine PubMed site at www.ncbi.nlm.nih.gov/pubmed/. You will see a box labeled "Search" with the term "PubMed" in it. The box next to it has the label "for" before it; type in "Nursing Research Survey Instruments." Click on "Go." Review the results you obtain.

    a. How many results were identified?

    b. Print the first page and review the first five citations. Do these citations give you information about the survey instruments that are available to use in nursing research?

    c. How is the information presented? Is it in a manner that is useful to planning research?

    d. How current is the information?

    e. Now place quotation marks around your search terms and search the following: nursing and research and "survey instruments." How many results were identified? Did the use of quotation marks make your search more targeted?

2. Now go to your library home page and choose a nursing database (CINAHL) or a general database (MEDLINE, Scopus, Ebsco). Access the database and open a search page. In the box, type in "Nursing Research Survey Instruments." Click on "search." Review the results you obtain.

    a. How many results were identified?

    b. Print the first page and review the first five citations. Do these citations differ from the first five citations on PubMed?

    c. How is the information presented? Is it in a manner that is useful to planning research?

    d. How current is the information?

Activity 7: Evidence-Based Practice Activity

1. What is the value of nonexperimental studies, such as ones that demonstrate a strong relationship in predictive correlational studies for evidence-based practice?
    a. None.
    b. They provide evidence only for training purposes.
    c. They demonstrate cause-and-effect relationships and can be used in decision making regarding changes in practice.
    d. They lend support for attempting to influence the independent variable in a future intervention study.

2. Which of the following nonexperimental designs provides a quality of evidence for evidence-based practice that is stronger than the others, because the researcher can determine the incidence of a problem and its possible causes?
    a. Cross-sectional
    b. Longitudinal cohort
    c. Survey

3. When you, the research consumer, are using the evidence-based practice model to consider a change in practice, you will initially make your decision based on the strength and quality of evidence provided by the meta-analysis. Following this, what other two characteristics will be important for you to consider? (There are two correct responses.)
    a. Clinical expertise
    b. Patient values
    c. The strength of the evidence
    d. The quality of the evidence
    e. The literature review

POSTTEST

Choose from among the following words to complete the posttest. Each word may be used one time; however, this list duplicates some words because they are used in more than one answer.

Comparative	Exploratory	Methodological	Retrospective
Correlational	Ex post facto	Prospective	Retrospective
Cross-sectional	Interrelational	Prospective	Survey
Cross-sectional	Longitudinal	Relationship-difference	Variables
Descriptive	Longitudinal	Retrospective	

1. In comparative surveys, the researcher does not manipulate the _____ but assesses data in order to provide data for future nursing intervention studies.

2. _____ is the broadest category of nonexperimental design.

3. The category from item 2 can be further classified as _____, _____, and _____.

4. The second major category of nonexperimental design according to LoBiondo-Wood and Haber includes _____ studies.

5. The researcher is using _____ design when examining the relationship between two or more variables.

6. _____ designs have many similarities to quasi-experimental designs.

7. _____ design used in epidemiological work is similar to ex post facto.

8. LoBiondo-Wood and Haber discuss three types of developmental studies. They are:

   a. _____

   b. _____

   c. _____

9. _____ studies collect data at one point in time while _____ collects data from the same group at different points in time.

10. A(n) _____ study looks at presumed causes and moves forward in time to presumed effects.

11. The researcher is using a _____ design if he or she is trying to link present events to events that have occurred in the past.

12. The _____ researcher is interested in identifying an intangible construct (concept) and making it tangible with a paper-and-pencil instrument or observation protocol.

REFERENCE

Rice VH, Stead LF: Nursing interventions for smoking cessation, *Cochrane Collaboration*, Issue 1, Hoboken, NJ, 2008, John Wiley & Sons.

Sampling

INTRODUCTION

Sampling is a process of selection in which individuals, objects, animals, or events are chosen to represent the population of a study. The ideal sampling strategy is one in which the elements truly represent the population being studied while controlling for any source of bias. The specific research question (or questions) determines the selection of the sample, variables to measure, and a sampling frame. The sampling strategies are important and should enable the choice of a sample that represents the target population and controls for bias as much as possible to ensure that the research will be valid. Reality modulates the ideal with the consideration of sampling in relation to efficiency, practicality, ethics, and availability of subjects, which can alter the ideal strategy for a given study.

LEARNING OUTCOMES

On completion of this chapter, the student should be able to do the following:

- Identify the purpose of sampling.
- Define *population, sample,* and *sampling.*
- Compare and contrast a population and a sample.
- Discuss the importance of inclusion and exclusion criteria for sample selection.
- Define *nonprobability* and *probability sampling.*
- Identify the types of nonprobability and probability sampling strategies.
- Compare the advantages and disadvantages of specific nonprobability and probability sampling strategies.
- Discuss the contribution of nonprobability and probability sampling strategies to strength of evidence provided by study findings.
- Discuss the factors that influence determination of sample size.
- Discuss the procedure for drawing a sample.
- Discuss potential threats to internal and external validity as sources of sampling bias.
- Use the critiquing criteria to evaluate the "Sample" section of a research report.

Activity 1

Write a short definition of each of the following and explain the differences among each set of words.

1. Sample _____

   Population _____

   Differences _____

2. Target Population _____

   Accessible Population _____

   Differences _____

3. Inclusion criteria _____

   Exclusion criteria _____

   Differences _____

Activity 2

1. Identify the key difference between probability and nonprobability sampling: _____
   _____

2. Identify the category of sampling for each of the following sampling strategies. Use the abbreviations from the key provided.

   Key:
   P = Probability sampling
   N = Nonprobability sampling

   a. _____   Convenience sampling

   b. _____   Purposive sampling

   c. _____   Simple random sampling

   d. _____   Quota sampling

   e. _____   Cluster sampling

   f. _____   Stratified random sampling

Activity 3

For each of the following examples of studies, identify the sampling strategy used from the following list. Write a letter that corresponds to the strategy in the space preceding the sampling description. Check the glossary for definition of terms.

    a. Convenience sampling
    b. Quota sampling
    c. Purposive sampling
    d. Simple random sampling
    e. Stratified random sampling

1. _____ The sample for the study of critical thinking behavior of undergraduate baccalaureate nursing students consisted of students enrolled in junior- and senior-level courses in three specific schools of nursing. In each program, students were invited to participate until a total sample representing 10% of the junior-level students and 10% of the senior-level students was obtained.

2. _____ Using a table of random numbers, the sample of 50 subjects was selected from a list of all mothers giving birth in the county during the first 6 months of the year.

3. _____ The sample was selected from residents of eight nursing homes in Arkansas and consisted of cognitively impaired people with no physical impairments or other psychiatric illness.

4. _____ The sample selected was parents who were chosen because of their knowledge and experience of having been a parent with a child in an NICU. Inclusion criteria included those parents with a child admitted to the NICU for more than a week, gestation at birth 26 weeks or above, on a ventilator for at least 3 days, and discharged home within the last 6 months.

5. _____ The sample consisted of adolescent mothers, meeting eligibility requirements, who were recruited from referrals to the Community Health Services Division of the County Health Department until the sample reached a target number of 144 participants. The mothers were randomly assigned using a computer-based program into one of two groups.

6. _____ To study the educational opportunities for nurses in various ethnic groups, a list of all nurses in the state of California was sorted by ethnicity. The sample consisted of 10% of the nurses in each ethnic group, selected according to a table of random numbers.

7. _____ A total of 155 infants were enrolled and divided into an intervention group of 72 infants and a control group of 83 infants. A computer program that generated random numbers made assignment to intervention or control group.

Activity 4

1. Refer to the study by Meneses et al. (2007) in Appendix A of your textbook.

    a. Is the sample adequately described?

        Yes   No

b. Do the sample characteristics correspond to the larger population?

Yes   No   Maybe

c. What sampling strategy was used in this study?

d. Is this a probability or nonprobability sample?

e. What was the sample size? What was the retention rate for subjects?

2. List one advantage of using the sampling strategy described in this study.

3. List one disadvantage of using the sampling strategy described in this study.

4. How does this sampling strategy support evidence in nursing practice?

Activity 5

Using the critical thinking decision path in the textbook, indicate whether the following statements are True (T) or False (F).

1. _____ Nonprobability sampling is associated with less generalizability to the larger population.

2. _____ Convenience sampling limits generalizability of findings largely because of the self-selection of subjects.

3. _____ Nonprobability sampling strategies are more time-consuming than probability strategies.

4. _____ Random sampling has the greatest risk of bias and is moderately representative.

5. _____ The easier the sampling strategy the greater the risk of bias, and as sampling becomes easier to implement, the risk of bias and limited representatives of the population increases.

6. _____ Purposive sampling procedures are the least generalizable sampling of the sampling strategies listed.

7. _____ Stratified random sampling uses a random selection procedure for obtaining sample subjects.

Activity 6

Review the following excerpt from a study. Using the critiquing criteria listed in the text, critique the sampling process used in this study. Refer to the study by Horgas, Yoon, Nichols, et al. (2008) (see Appendix C).

A convenience sample was recruited from five senior centers and two churches in a large, racially diverse city in the Midwest in 2000. All seniors present in the facility on the day of the survey were invited to participate. Inclusion criteria were: ≥60 years old, willing to participate, and able to provide informed consent. Ability to consent was ascertained by explaining the study to potential participants, who were then asked to describe the study. Participants were excluded if they were unable to explain the study and provide consent or were unable to complete the survey. Because this was a community-based, volunteer sample, very few participants were excluded on this basis (approximately 5% of participants who expressed interest in the study was unable to consent or complete the survey). A total of 115 community-dwelling older adults completed the survey. The sample was predominantly female, had an age range of 62–95 years, and was almost equally divided between Black and White older adults (see Table 1). As shown in Table 1, Blacks and Whites differed significantly in several sociodemographic and health variables. Black participants were generally older; more likely to be female, unmarried, and have lower levels of education and income; and more Blacks suffered from functionally limiting medical conditions than Whites in this sample. Thus, these variables were included as covariates in the statistical analyses.

1. Have the sample characteristics been completely described? (Explain your answer.)

2. Can the parameters of the study population be inferred from the description of the sample?

3. To what extent is the sample representative of the population as defined?

4. Are criteria for eligibility in the sample specifically identified?

5. Have sample delimitations been established? (Explain your answer.)

6. Would it be possible to replicate the study sample? (Explain your answer.)

7. How was the sample selected? Is the method of sample selection appropriate?

8. What kind of bias, if any, is introduced by this method?

9. Is the sample size appropriate? How is it substantiated?

10. Are there indications that the rights of the subjects have been ensured?

11. Do the researchers identify the limitations in generalizability of the findings from the sample to the population? Are they appropriate?

Activity 7: Web-Based Activity

Go to the U.S. Census website at www.census.gov. Click on "Find an Area Profile with Quick Facts" at the bottom right-hand corner of the screen. In the box where it asks you, "To begin, select a state from this list or use the map to your right," select your home state from the drop-down menu. Click on the "Go" button.

1. Under your state's Quick Facts, look at the item titled "White persons, percent" and write down that percent.

2. Now look for the item titled "Black persons, percent" and write down that percent.

3. How are these groups defined? (Hint: Click on the *i* on the left side of the screen.)

4. Now go back to Activity 5. Review the sample percents in the Horgas et al. (2008) study for white and black people; are they the same as they are in the census data? Would the sample percents for black and white in the Horgas et al. study be representative of the population in your state?

Activity 8: Evidence-Based Practice Activity

The text defines *evidence-based practice* (EBP) as the integration of best research evidence with clinical expertise and patient values. EBP allows nurses to utilize research findings to make decisions to improve practice. Teams of nurses are applying multiple study findings to improve practice outcomes with individuals, families, and other health care professionals. Through this practice, more effective patient teaching and quality care are being realized.

What is the relationship between sampling and evidence-based practice decision making? In other words, how will the sampling strategy in a study or a meta-analysis of studies influence how you and your colleagues make a decision about changing the practice in your health care setting? (Hint: Review the five Evidence-Based Practice Tips in Chapter 10 before answering this question.)

POSTTEST

Complete the sentences below.

1. A statistical technique known as _____ may be used to determine sample size in quantitative studies.

2. Sampling strategies are grouped into two categories: _____ sampling and _____ sampling.

3. _____ sampling is the use of the most readily accessible people or objects as subjects in a study.

4. Advantages of _____ sampling are low bias and maximal representativeness, but the disadvantage is the labor in drawing a sample.

5. A(n) _____ can be used to select an unbiased sample or unbiased assignment of subjects to treatment groups.

6. A(n) _____ sample is one whose key characteristics closely approximate those of the population.

7. _____ criteria are used to select the sample from all possible units and _____ may be used to restrict the population to a homogenous group of subjects.

8. Types of nonprobability sampling include _____, _____, and _____ sampling.

9. Successive random sampling of units that progress from large to small and meet sample eligibility criteria is known as _____ sampling.

10. In certain qualitative studies, subjects are added to the sample until _____ occurs (new data no longer emerge during data collection).

REFERENCES

Horgas AL, Yoon SL, Nichols AL, et al.: The relationship between pain and functional disability in black and white older adults, *Res Nurs Health* 31(4):341-354, 2008.

Meneses DK, McNees P, Loerzel W, et al.: Transition from treatment to survivorship: effects of a psychoeducational intervention on quality of life in breast cancer survivors, *Oncol Nurs Forum* 34:1007-1016, 2007.

U.S. Census Bureau: Retrieved August, 26, 2009, from www.census.gov.

Legal and Ethical Issues

INTRODUCTION

Patient advocacy is one of the primary roles of a professional nurse. Nowhere is this more important than in the field of research. The nurse must be a patient advocate, whether acting as the researcher, a participant in data gathering, a provider of care for research subjects, or a research consumer. A multitude of legal and ethical issues exist in research; nurses must be aware of, assess, act on, and evaluate these issues. In addition, nurses need to be knowledgeable about the purpose and functions of the institutional review board (IRB) and the federal regulations on which they are based.

LEARNING OUTCOMES

On completion of this chapter, the student should be able to do the following:

- Describe the historical background that led to the development of ethical guidelines for the use of human subjects in research.
- Identify the essential elements of an informed consent form.
- Evaluate the adequacy of an informed consent form.
- Describe the institutional review board's role in the research review process.
- Identify populations of subjects who require special legal and ethical research considerations.
- Appreciate the nurse researcher's obligations to conduct and report research in an ethical manner.
- Describe the nurse's role as patient advocate in research situations.
- Critique the ethical aspects of a research study.

Activity 1

Fill in the blanks with the correct term from the following list (you do not need to use all of the terms):

Beneficence   Justice
Confidentiality   Nursing research committee
Expedited review   Unauthorized research
Institutional review board   Unethical research study
HIPAA

1. _____ reviews proposals for scientific merit and congruence with the institutional policies and missions.

2. _____ reviews research proposals to ensure protection of the rights of human subjects.

3. The idea that human subjects should be treated fairly and should not be denied a benefit to which the subject is entitled is _____.

4. A study of existing data that is of minimal risk to subjects may be a candidate for a(n) _____.

5. The U.S. Public Health Service studied the effects of untreated syphilis on African-American sharecroppers in Tuskegee, Alabama and withheld penicillin treatment even after penicillin was commonly available. This is considered a(n) _____.

6. Regulation requires the health care profession to protect privacy of patient information and create standards for electronic data exchange _____.

Activity 2

List the three ethical principles relevant to the conduct of research involving human subjects. These were included in the Belmont Report (1979) and formed the basis for regulations affecting research sponsored by the federal government.

1. _____

2. _____

3. _____

Activity 3

Read the following example of a research consent form. Then review the list of the elements of informed consent that follows the example. For each item in the list of elements of informed consent, put either a "✓" if the element is included in the consent or a "0" if it is absent from the consent. Summarize your findings in a paragraph at the end of the exercise.

Research Consent Form
Agreement to Participate in Research

Responsible Investigator: Serena Anderson, PhD, Professor, Nursing

Title of Protocol: A Web-based interactive program to engage nurses in learning principles of pain management.

We are recruiting nursing students to test a Web-based interactive program to engage nurses in learning principles of pain management. There are three learning outcomes for this program, to teach the following: (1) appropriate and safe control of the patient's pain, (2) prevention and management of side effects of pain management, and (3) to provide accurate and complete patient teaching regarding pain and side effect management. At the end of the simulation, you will receive three scores, one for how well you managed patient care in each of these areas. It will take about 30 minutes to complete the simulation. The simulation is available online at www.cdl.edu/painless. You can complete the simulation as many times as you like; each time you will be presented with a new set of variables for the patient, Mr. Sanchez. The variables are programmed to appear randomly. We hope that this activity will enhance your knowledge related to providing pain management for your patients. There are no known risks for participation.

If you agree to participate, we welcome you and would like you to complete a pretest and posttest, as well as a short evaluation form after you complete the simulation. Your participation is voluntary, and you may withdraw at any time and for any reason. There is no penalty for not participating or for withdrawing. The personal benefits for participation include assisting faculty and yourself to understand more about the effectiveness of this innovative educational intervention and to increase your knowledge. There are no costs to you or any other party.

I will ask you to print a copy of your scores from the simulation, and complete the pretest and posttest and a short questionnaire. All data collected will be coded using a unique five-character string and will not be identified with you personally. There is no risk to you.

Dr. Serena Anderson, Professor, School of Nursing, San Jose State University is conducting this study. Dr. Anderson can be reached at 408-555-1000. You should understand that your participation is voluntary and that choosing not to participate in this study, or in any part of this study, will not affect your relations with San Jose State University. You may refuse to participate in the entire study or in any part of the study; you are free to withdraw at any time without any negative effect on your relations with San Jose State University. The results of this study may be published, but any information that could result in your identification will remain confidential. If you have questions about this study, I will be happy to talk with you. I can be reached at 408-555-1000. If you have questions or complaints about research subjects' rights, or in the event of a research-related injury, please contact Amy Smith, PhD, Associate Vice President for Graduate Studies and Research, at 408-555-1000.

This project has been reviewed and approved according to the San Jose State University Human Subjects Institutional Review Board procedures governing human subjects research.

Your signature indicates that you have been fully informed of your rights and voluntarily agree to participate in this study. You will be given a copy of this signed form. By signing this form, I agree to participate in this study.

_____   _____

Subject's Signature   Date

Elements of Informed Consent

1. _____   Title of protocol

2. _____   Invitation to participate

3. _____   Basis for subject selection

4. _____   Overall purpose of the study

5. _____   Explanation of benefits

6. _____   Description of risks and discomforts

7. _____   Potential benefits

8. _____   Alternatives to participation

9. _____   Financial obligations

10. _____   Assurance of confidentiality

11. _____   In case of injury compensation

12. _____   HIPAA disclosure

13. _____   Subject withdrawal

14. _____   Offer to answer questions

15. _____   Concluding consent statement

16. _____   Identification of investigators

Activity 4

Nurses must be aware of populations who require special legal and ethical considerations. List at least four groups of subjects who are vulnerable or have diminished autonomy and thus require extra protection as research subjects.

1. _____

2. _____

3. _____

4. _____

Activity 5

Match the violation of ethical principle described from the following list with the examples presented below. More than one violation may have occurred in the examples that are cited. List all that were violated.

    a. Degree of risk outweighed benefits
    b. Subjects not informed they could withdraw from study at any time
    c. Subjects not informed or offered the effective treatment that was available
    d. Lack of informed consent
    e. No evidence of IRB approval before start of research
    f. Right to fair treatment and protection
    g. Principles of informed consent violated or incomplete disclosure of potential risk, harm, results, or side effects was not given

1. Write the letter(s) describing violation after the description of the study.

   UCLA Schizophrenic Medication Study—a 1983 study examining the effects of withdrawing psychotropic medications of 50 patients under treatment for schizophrenia. Twenty-three subjects suffered severe relapses after their medications were stopped. The goal of the study was to determine if some schizophrenics might do better without medications that had deleterious side effects. Patients were not informed that their symptoms could worsen or about the severity of a potential relapse. _____

2. List the letter(s) that corresponds to the ethical violation(s) listed.

   The United States Public Health Service conducted a study from 1932 to 1973 on two groups of poor African-American male sharecroppers. One group had untreated syphilis and the other did not. Treatment was withheld from the group diagnosed with syphilis, even after it became generally available and known to be effective. Steps were taken to prevent infected subjects from obtaining penicillin. The researchers wanted to study the effects of untreated syphilis. _____

Activity 6

This activity assesses the utilization of procedures for protecting basic human rights. Review the articles in Appendices A through D of the text. For each article, describe how informed consent was obtained, and whether the authors described obtaining permission from the institutional review board.

1. Meneses et al. (2007):

2. Horgas et al. (2008):

3. Jones et al. (2007):

4. Landreneau et al. (2007):

Activity 7: Web-Based Activity

Go to the website www.cancer.gov.

1. Identify the source of this website.

2. Is this a reputable source that would provide reliable and valid information to inform a nursing practice?

Yes, because

No, because

Click on "Clinical Trials" at the top. Scroll down and click on "Conducting Clinical Trials." At the left, select "Participants in Clinical Trials," then click on the link "Clinical Research Training for Members of the Research Team at the NIH Clinical Center." Next, click on the link to www.nihtraining.com/cc/crt/indexvideo.html. Fill in the registration information with a user name and password of your choice. Review the tutorial and complete the online quiz to determine your comprehension of this material. The NIH now requires education in the protection of human research participants for all investigators and key personnel submitting NIH applications for grants or proposals for contracts, or receiving new or noncompeting awards. You may complete this program if you like, or if your instructor requires it. If you complete all the tutorials successfully, print the certificate and add this item to your résumé.

Activity 8: Evidence-Based Practice Activity

You are a nurse working in a postpartum unit. If you decided to make a change in your practice based on an evidence-based practice article, but first wanted to check to be certain that no misconduct had occurred in the conduct or reporting of the study, where would you find this information?

POSTTEST

1. It is necessary for researchers and nurses to protect the basic human rights of vulnerable groups. Can research studies be conducted with these populations?

Yes, because

No, because

2. A researcher must receive IRB approval (before, after) beginning to conduct research involving humans.

3. If you question whether a researcher has permission to conduct a study in your hospital, which documents would you want to see that demonstrate approval from which group(s)?

_____

4. Should a researcher list all the possible risks and benefits of a participating in a research study even if some people may refuse because these items are listed in detail?

   Yes   No

5. If you agreed to collect data for a researcher who had not asked the patient's permission to participate in the research study, you would be violating the patient's right to

   _____.

6. What are two of the risks of scientific fraud or misconduct?

REFERENCES

Horgas AL, Yoon SL, Nichols AL, et al.: The relationship between pain and functional disability in black and white older adults, *Res Nurs Health* 31(4):341-354, 2008.

Jones EG, Renger R, Kang Y: Self-efficacy for health-related behaviors among deaf adults, *Res Nurs Health* 30:185-192, 2007.

Landreneau KJ, Ward-Smith P: Perceptions of adult patients on hemodialysis concerning choice among renal replacement therapies, *Nephrol Nurs* 34(5):513-519, 525, 2007.

Meneses DK, McNees P, Loerzel W, et al.: Transition from treatment to survivorship: Effects of a psychoeducational intervention on quality of life in breast cancer survivors, *Oncol Nurs Forum* 34:1007-1016, 2007.

National Cancer Institute: Retrieved August 26, 2009, from www.cancer.gov.

12

Data-Collection Methods

INTRODUCTION

Observe, probe
Details unfold
Let nature's secrets
Be stammeringly retold.

> —*Goethe*

The focus of this chapter is basic information about data collection. As a consumer of research, the reader needs the skills to evaluate and critique data-collection methods in published research studies. In order to achieve these skills, it is helpful to have an appreciation of the process or the critical thinking "journey" the researcher has taken to be ready to collect the data. Each of the preceding chapters represented important preliminary steps in the research planning and designing phases before data collection. Although most researchers are eager to begin data collection, the planning for data collection is very important. The planning includes identifying and prioritizing data needs, developing or selecting appropriate data-collection tools, and selecting and training data-collection personnel before proceeding with actual collection of data.

The five types of data-collection methods differ in their basic approach and the strengths and weaknesses of their characteristics. Readers should be prepared to ask questions about the appropriateness of the measures chosen by the researcher to gather data about the variable of concern. This includes determining the objectivity, consistency, quantifiability, observer intervention, and/or obtrusiveness of the chosen data-collection method.

LEARNING OUTCOMES

On completion of this chapter, the reader should be able to do the following:

- Define the types of data-collection methods used in nursing research.
- List the advantages and disadvantages of each data-collection method.
- Compare how specific data-collection methods contribute to the strength of evidence in a research study.
- Identify potential sources of bias related to data collection.
- Discuss the importance of intervention fidelity in data collection.
- Critically evaluate the data-collection methods used in published research studies.

Activity 1

Review each of the articles referenced below. Be especially thorough in reading the sections that relate to data-collection methods. Answer the questions in relation to what you understand from the article. For some questions, there may be more than one answer.

Study 1

Meneses et al. (2007) (in Appendix A of the text).

1. Which data-collection method(s) is/are used in this research study?
   a. A physiological measure
   b. An observational measure
   c. An interview measure
   d. A questionnaire measure
   e. Records of available data

2. In your opinion, what would be the advantage in using this method(s)? What explanation do the investigators provide?

Study 2

Jones et al. (2007) (in Appendix B of the text).

1. Which data-collection method is used in this research study?
   a. A physiological measure
   b. An observational measure
   c. An interview measure
   d. A questionnaire
   e. Records of available data

2. Rationale for appropriateness of data-collection method:

3. What is your opinion as to the success of the method chosen?

Study 3

Horgas et al. (2008) (in Appendix C of the text).

1. What data-collection method is used in this research study?
   a. A physiological measure
   b. An observational measure
   c. An interview measure
   d. A questionnaire
   e. Records of available data

2. What were the strengths in using this method?

Study 4

Landreneau et al. (2007) (in Appendix D of the text).

1. What data-collection method is used in this research study?
    a. A physiological measure
    b. An observational measure
    c. An interview measure
    d. A questionnaire
    e. Records of available data

2. What are two possible problems with self-report methods that might have affected the re-sponses given by participants? Are there ways for researchers to prevent these problems?

Activity 2

Using the content of Chapter 12 in the text, have fun with the word search exercise. Answer the questions below and find the words in the puzzle.

1. Baccalaureate-prepared nurses are _____ of research.

2. _____ are those methods that use technical instruments to collect data about patients' physical, chemical, microbiological, or anatomical status.

3. _____ is the distortion of data as a result of the observer's presence.

4. _____ are best used when a large response rate and an unbiased sample are important.

5. _____ data-collection method is subject to problems of availability, authenticity, and accuracy.

6. _____ measurements are especially useful when there are a finite number of questions to be asked and the questions are clear and specific.

7. Essential in the critique of data-collection methods is the emphasis on the appropriateness, _____, and _____ of the method employed.

8. _____ raises ethical questions (especially informed consent issues); therefore it is not often used in nursing.

9. _____ _____ is the consistency of observations between two or more observers.

10. _____ is the process of translating the concepts/variables into measurable phenomena.

11. _____ is a format that uses close-ended items, and there are a fixed number of alternative responses.

12. _____ is the method for objective, systematic, and quantitative description of communications and documentary evidence.

13. This exercise is supposed to be _____!

```
D  E  L  I  V  E  R  S  T  A  T  I  S  T  C  S  Y  E  S  P  A  S
S  S  A  C  A  B  I  N  E  T  F  O  R  K  A  Z  O  S  P  E  I  O
I  A  W  O  P  E  R  A  T  I  O  N  A  L  I  Z  A  T  I  O  N  B
G  T  S  N  O  R  N  E  V  E  R  B  Y  D  N  E  A  U  X  B  T  J
N  S  Y  S  T  E  M  A  T  I  C  A  J  H  T  B  S  D  V  S  E  E
I  F  L  I  K  E  R  T  S  C  A  L  E  E  R  R  O  Y  A  E  R  C
F  A  K  S  C  A  L  E  S  N  O  V  N  O  C  A  A  U  L  R  R  T
H  C  U  T  A  C  R  A  T  I  M  A  P  V  E  T  P  U  I  V  A  I
Y  T  B  E  B  H  I  R  T  E  M  A  H  V  W  K  I  C  D  A  T  V
P  C  O  N  T  E  N  T  A  N  A  L  Y  S  I  S  P  V  O  T  E  I
R  O  Y  C  B  K  D  S  I  S  R  T  S  A  D  V  A  N  E  I  R  T
E  R  E  Y  O  D  U  G  K  A  T  P  I  B  I  O  I  O  G  O  R  Y
A  V  S  I  B  R  Q  U  E  S  T  I  O  N  N  A  I  R  E  N  E  C
C  I  A  R  E  S  E  A  R  C  H  L  L  R  E  A  C  E  S  O  L  O
T  O  B  M  E  X  C  E  L  A  E  O  O  D  A  T  A  C  O  V  I  N
I  U  E  A  E  V  A  L  I  D  S  T  G  N  O  S  T  O  O  E  A  S
V  N  Y  E  S  S  I  N  T  E  R  V  I  E  W  S  A  R  F  R  B  U
I  H  A  P  P  I  E  N  E  S  S  P  C  A  T  A  G  D  U  N  I  M
T  X  C  I  T  E  D  E  L  P  H  I  A  T  O  T  P  S  N  V  L  E
Y  C  E  A  T  U  B  B  S  A  N  D  L  D  O  N  N  M  A  R  I  R
Y  A  B  L  E  A  C  O  N  C  E  A  L  M  E  N  T  O  O  T  T  R
A  I  K  E  V  A  L  I  K  E  I  I  A  B  C  O  N  S  U  M  Y  S
```

Activity 3

You are reviewing a study, and concealment is necessary; in other words, there is no other way to collect the data, and the data collected will not have negative consequences for the subject.

1. Name at least one population where concealment is not uncommon.

2. How would you obtain subjects' consent?

3. What is the major reason for using concealment?

Activity 4

You are asked to participate in discussions about impending research in your community. The purpose of the study is to identify the health status, beliefs, practices, preventive services currently known and used, and accessibility/availability of health service needs for the residents of your rural community.

In your critical thinking journey, describe what you would consider in the selection of a data-collection method. Review each method and discuss the pros and cons for choosing a specific data-collection method. State your rationale for your final selection. What would be your thinking about instruments and types?

Activity 5

Using the content of Chapter 12 in the textbook, circle the correct response for each question. Some questions will have more than one answer.

1. What is a primary advantage of physiological measures?
    a. The measuring tool never affects the phenomena being measured
    b. It is one of the easiest types of methods to implement
    c. It is unlikely that study participants/subjects can distort the physiological information
    d. Their objectivity, sensitivity, and precision
    e. All of the above

2. Self-report measures are usually more useful than observation measures in obtaining information about which of the following?
    a. Socially unacceptable or private behaviors
    b. Complex research situations when it is difficult to separate processes and interactions
    c. When the researcher is interested in character traits
    d. All of the above

3. Which of the following would be considered disadvantages of using observational data-collection methods?
    a. Individual bias may interfere with the data collection
    b. Ethical concerns may be increasingly significant to researchers using observational data-collection methods
    c. Individual judgments and values influence the perceptions of the observers
    d. All of the above

4. In nursing research, when might questionnaires be used as an appropriate method for data collection?
    a. Whenever expense is a concern for the researcher
    b. When a researcher is interested in obtaining information directly from the subjects
    c. When the researcher needs to collect data from a large group of subjects who are not easily accessible
    d. When accuracy is of the utmost importance to the researcher

5. Which of the following would be considered advantages of using existing records or available data to answer a research question?
   a. The use of available data reduces the risk of researcher bias in data collection
   b. Time involvement in the research study can be reduced by the use of available records or data
   c. Consistent collection of information over periods of time allows the researcher to study trends
   d. All of the above

Activity 6: Web-Based Activity

Go to your library home page. Select your favorite database (some to try: PubMed, Scopus, CINAHL, MEDLINE). Open the database and search for the following terms: "nursing assessment" AND tool AND development.

How many nursing-specific assessment tools can you identify in the first 20 citations? What was the focus of the different tools? Did you see any tools you are familiar with?

Now choose an area of nursing that you are interested in and search for data measurement tools in that area. Some potential topics include fall prevention, pressure ulcers, depression, infection, anxiety, quality of life, pain, and satisfaction.

Activity 7: Evidence-Based Practice Activity

Check the evidence-based practice resources available at your clinical site or go to your library home page. Find the Cochrane Library or any database with access to evidence-based resources. Search for the term "nursing intervention." Choose a recent study of a nursing intervention you might use in your practice.

1. What were some of the methods used in studies included in this review? Were the methods appropriate?

2. Would you change your practice based on the evidence provided in this study? Explain your answer.

3. After looking at the "Results" and "Discussion" sections of the article you reviewed, how would you improve the data collection methods of the studies under review to strengthen the evidence?

POSTTEST

Read each question thoroughly and then circle the correct answer.

1. What is the process of translating concepts that are of interest to the researcher into observable and measurable phenomena?
    a. Objectivism
    b. Systematization
    c. Subjectivism
    d. Operationalization

2. Research questions pertaining to psychosocial variables can best be answered by using which data-gathering technique(s)?
    a. Observation
    b. Interviews
    c. Questionnaires
    d. All of the above

3. Collection of data from each subject in the same or in a similar manner is known as:
    a. Repetition
    b. Dualism
    c. Consistency
    d. Recidivism

4. Consistency of observations between two or more observers is known as:
    a. Intrarater reliability
    b. Interrater reliability
    c. Consistency reliability
    d. Repetitive reliability

5. Physiological and biological measurement might be used by nurse researchers when studying which of these variables? (Select all that apply.)
    a. A comparison of student nurses' ACT scores and their GPAs
    b. Hypertensive clients' responses to a stress test
    c. Children's dietary patterns
    d. The degree of pain relief achieved following guided imagery

6. Scientific observations should fulfill which of the following conditions?
    a. Observations are consistent with the study objectives.
    b. Observations are standardized and systematically recorded.
    c. Observations are checked and controlled.
    d. All of the above

7. In a research study, a participant observer spent regularly scheduled hours in a homeless shelter and occasionally stayed overnight. The people staying in the home were told that this person was conducting a research study. The researcher freely engaged in conversation and openly observed the homeless. What is the observational role of the researcher?
    a. Concealment without intervention
    b. Concealment with intervention
    c. No concealment without intervention
    d. No concealment with intervention

8. In unstructured observation, which of the following might occur? (Select all that apply.)
   a. Extensive field notes are recorded.
   b. Subjects are informed what behaviors are being observed.
   c. The researcher frequently records interesting anecdotes.
   d. All of the above

9. Which of the following is not consistent with a Likert scale?
   a. It contains close-ended items.
   b. It contains open-ended items.
   c. It contains lists of statements.
   d. Items are evaluated on the amount of agreement.

10. Although it is acceptable to use multiple instruments within a research study, the study is more acceptable if only one method is used for the data collection.
    a. True
    b. False

11. Social desirability is seldom a concern for researchers when the data-collection method used in the study is interviews.
    a. True
    b. False

12. A researcher wants to use a questionnaire in a study but cannot find one that will gather the information desired about a particular variable. The decision is made to develop a new instrument. Which of the following should the researcher do?
    a. Define the construct, formulate the items, and assess the items for content validity
    b. Develop instructions for users and pilot the instrument
    c. Estimate reliability and validity
    d. All of the above

13. The researcher who invests significant amounts of time in the development of an instrument has a professional responsibility to publish the results.
    a. True
    b. False

14. In order to evaluate the adequacy of various data-collection methods, which of the following should be observed in the written research report?
    a. Clear identification of the rationale for selecting a physiological measure
    b. The problems of bias and reactivity are addressed with observational measures
    c. There is a clear explanation of how interviews were conducted and how interviewers were trained
    d. All of the above

15. In conducting a research study, the researcher has a responsibility to ensure that all study subjects received the same information and data were collected from all participants in the same manner.
    a. True
    b. False

REFERENCES

Horgas AL, Yoon SL, Nichols AL, et al.: The relationship between pain and functional disability in black and white older adults, *Res Nurs Health* 31(4):341-354, 2008.

Jones EG, Renger R, Kang Y: Self-efficacy for health-related behaviors among deaf adults, *Res Nurs Health* 30:185-192, 2007.

Landreneau KJ, Ward-Smith P: Perceptions of adult patients on hemodialysis concerning choice among renal replacement therapies, *Nephrol Nurs* 34(5):513-519, 525, 2007.

Meneses DK, McNees P, Loerzel W, et al.: Transition from treatment to survivorship: Effects of a psychoeducational intervention on quality of life in breast cancer survivors, *Oncol Nurs Forum* 34:1007-1016, 2007.

13

Reliability and Validity

INTRODUCTION

If someone tells you, "Hey, I found a new restaurant that you will really love," you will consider that information from at least two perspectives before you spend your money there. First, does this person know what she is talking about when it comes to your taste in food? Second, has this person given you good information about food in the past?

You answer "no" to the first question. You prefer seafood served in an elegant setting, and your friend prefers pizza served in a place with sawdust on the floor. Using this information, you will consider her opinion to be invalid for you. You will never give this restaurant another thought.

But if you answer "yes" to the first question because you share similar tastes in food, you will move on to the second question. You remember the tough fettuccini, the subpar Southern fried chicken, the unbaked pizza dough, and the hockey-puck biscuits from earlier recommendations. It is likely that while you and your friend share food preferences, her information is not reliable. You can't trust her to give you good information over time. If you are feeling like an adventure, you may try the new restaurant or you may not.

Validity and reliability of the data-collection instruments used in a study are to be regarded in the same way that you would consider your friend's advice about restaurants. Is the instrument valid? Does it provide me with accurate information? Is the instrument reliable? Does it provide me with consistent information whenever it is used? Consideration of both validity and reliability influences your confidence in the results of the study.

LEARNING OUTCOMES

On completion of this chapter, the student should be able to do the following:

- Discuss how measurement error can affect the outcomes of a research study.
- Discuss the purposes of reliability and validity.
- Define *reliability*.
- Discuss the concepts of stability, equivalence, and homogeneity as they relate to reliability.
- Compare and contrast the estimates of reliability.
- Define *validity*.
- Compare and contrast content, criterion-related, and construct validity.
- Identify the criteria for critiquing the reliability and validity of measurement tools.
- Use the critiquing criteria to evaluate the reliability and validity of measurement tools.
- Discuss how evidence related to reliability and validity contributes to the strength and quality of evidence provided by the findings of a research study and applicability to practice.

Activity 1

Either random error (*R*) or systematic error (*S*) may occur in a research study. For each of the following examples, identify the type of measurement error and how the error might be corrected.

1. _____   The scale used to obtain daily weights was inaccurate by 3 pounds less than actual weight.

   Correction:

2. _____   Students chose the socially acceptable responses on an instrument to assess attitudes toward AIDS patients.

   Correction:

3. _____   Confusion existed among the evaluators on how to score the wound healing.

   Correction:

4. _____   The subjects were nervous about taking the psychological tests.

   Correction:

Activity 2

Validity is the extent to which a measurement tool actually measures the concepts it is supposed to measure. Use the terms from the following list to complete each of the items in this activity.

Concurrent validity	Content validity	Contrasted groups
Construct validity	Convergent validity	Criterion-related validity
Divergent validity	Content validity index	Factor analysis
Hypothesis testing	Multitrait-multimethod approach	Predictive validity
Rating from a panel of experts		

1. _____of the instrument was evaluated by exploratory factor analysis (EFA) and confirmatory factor analysis (CFA). Samples sizes for EFA and CFA were 632 and 578, respectively.

2. _____ is an intuitive, preliminary type of instrument evaluation. Does the instrument appear to measure the concept?

3. "This measure has been found to be a reliable and valid measure of pain intensity, and it has demonstrated _____ with other pain intensity scales" (Horgas et al., 2008).

4. The survey design process began with occupational health nurses who told the authors and graduate nursing students what information they sought from the survey. The authors and

six doctoral students used these ideas to develop a one-page questionnaire titled "Travel Health." The occupational health nurses ($n = 10$) served as _____. They reviewed and revised the survey before it was sent to the international business center for final approval.

5. The current study showed that when the Fatigue Symptom Scale and the TIRED Scale were given to the same subjects and a correlational analysis was performed, there was _____ based on the positive correlation between both measures of the concept of fatigue.

6. Construct validity, an assessment of the relationship between the instrument and the underlying theory, can be measured in several ways. List three of these: _____, _____, and _____.

7. An instrument is being developed to measure physical activity in knee injury patients. The instrument was administered to a group of patients the day before surgery and another group of patients 6 months after surgery. A t-test found significant differences between the groups. This is a _____ test of construct validity.

Activity 3

An instrument is considered reliable if it is accurate and consistent. If the concept being studied is stable, the same results should occur when measurement is repeated.

1. Three concepts related to reliability include _____, _____, and _____.

2. Give an example of each of the two types of tests for stability.

3. In what instance would it be better to use an alternate form rather than a test-retest measure for stability?

4. Homogeneity is a measure of internal consistency. All items on the instrument should be complementary and measure the same characteristic or concepts. For each of the following examples, identify which of the following tests for homogeneity is described:

(1) Item-total correlations
(2) Split-half reliability
(3) Kuder-Richardson (KR-20) coefficient
(4) Cronbach's alpha

a. _____ The odd items of the test had a high correlation with the even numbers of the test.

b. _____ Each item on the test using a 5-point Likert scale had a moderate correlation with every other item on the test.

c. _____ Each item on the test ranged in correlation from 0.62 to 0.89 with the total.

d. _____ Each item on the true-false test had a moderate correlation with every other item on the test.

5. Review the information about one of the instruments used in the Horgas et al. (2008) study in Appendix C of the text.

> The SIP Short Form (SIP68), one of the most widely used generic measures of health-related functioning, was used to measure physical and social disability. The SIP, originally developed as a broad measure of health-related behavior (Bergner, Bobbit, Carter, & Gilson, 1981), was reported to be valid and reliable (de Bruin, de Witte, Stevens, & Diederiks, 1992), but it was considered to be too lengthy and burdensome for some older adults to complete. The SIP68 has 68 items with 6 subscales: somatic autonomy, mobility control, psychic autonomy, and communication (mental functioning and verbal communication), social behavior, emotional stability, and mobility range.

a. Think about the concept of face validity. Think about the variables being addressed in the study. Would you conclude that these instruments had face validity for this study?

b. What information is given to the reader about the SIP?

c. How does this information influence your level of confidence in the results of this study?

Activity 4: Web-Based Activity

Go to www.cdc.gov. Click on "A-Z Index" (at the top of the page). Click on "H," then scroll down to "Health-Related Quality of Life," then to "Methods and Measures." Scroll to "Measurement Properties" and click. Scroll through to find a full-text link to an article, and click on it. Read the first part of the article.

1. How does the CDC measure health-related quality of life?

2. Find the studies on validity and reliability. What are some other measures of health-related quality of life that the CDC HRQOL has been compared to?

Activity 5

In this activity you will use the critiquing criteria listed in Chapter 13 of the text to think about the Meneses et al. (2007) study in Appendix A of the text.

1. How many instruments for data collection were used in this study?

2. For the Quality of Life–Breast Cancer Survivors scale:

a. What information on validity was included in the article?

b. What methods were used to test reliability?

c. Was the reliability of the instrument adequate?

d. Was the reliability calculated for this study population?

e. How did the researchers minimize threats to internal and external reliability?

f. Do the authors discuss the threats to validity in the study?

Activity 6: Evidence-Based Practice Activity

Now think about the study reviewed in Activity 5. Look at the table you have completed regarding the reliability and validity measures of the instruments used in the study. Assume you are a nurse in oncology. How would you use the results of this study to guide your practice?

POSTTEST

Using the following terms, complete the sentences for the type of validity or reliability discussed. Terms may be used more than once.

Content	Test-retest
Factor analysis	Cronbach's alpha
Convergent	Alternate or parallel form
Divergent	Interrater
Concurrent	

1. In tests for reliability, the self-efficacy scale had a(n) _____ of 0.88, demonstrating internal consistency for the new measure.

2. The ABC social support scale demonstrated _____ validity with correlation of 0.84 with the XYZ interpersonal relationships scale.

3. _____ validity was supported with a correlation of 0.42 between the ABC social support scale and the QRS loneliness scale.

4. The investigator established _____ validity through evaluation of the cardiac recovery scale by a panel of cardiac clinical nurse specialists. All items were rated 0 to 5 for importance to recovery and only items scoring above an average of 3 were kept in the final scale.

5. The results of the _____ were that all the items clustered around three factors, lending support to the notion that there are three dimensions of coping.

6. The observations were rated by three experts. The _____ reliability among the observers was 94%.

7. To assess _____ reliability, subjects completed the locus of control questionnaire at the beginning of the project and 2 weeks later. The correlation of 0.86 supports the stability of the concept.

8. Bennett et al. (1996) developed an instrument called the Cardiac Event Threat Questionnaire (CTQ). They established _____ validity by reviewing the literature reviewing concerns identified by patients recovering from a cardiac event, and had the items critiqued by a panel of experts.

9. The results of the CTQ that measured threat were highly correlated with the results of a test measuring negative emotions. This established _____ validity.

10. Bennett et al. (1996) reported that internal consistency reliabilities of the five factors of the CTQ were computed with the _____ statistic.

REFERENCES

Bennett SJ et al. (1996). Development of an instrument to measure threat related to cardiac events, *Nurs Res* 45:266–270.

Bergner M, Bobbit RA, Carter WB, Gilson BS (1981). The Sickness Impact Profile: Development and final evaluation of a health status measure. *Medical Care*, 19, 787–805.

de Bruin AF, de Witte LP, Stevens F, Diedericks JPM (1992). Sickness Impact Profile: The state of the art of a generic functional status measure. *Social Science and Medicine*, 35, 1003–1014.

Horgas AL, Yoon SL, Nichols AL, Marsiske M: The relationship between pain and functional disability in black and white older adults, *Res Nurs Health* (40):341-354, 2008.

Meneses KD, McNees P, Loerzel VW, et al.: Transition from treatment to survivorship: Effects of a psychoeducational intervention on quality of life in breast cancer survivors, *Oncol Nurs Forum* 34(5):1007-1016, 2007.

U.S. Department of Health and Human Services: Centers for Disease Control. Retrieved August 27, 2009, from www.cdc.gov/.

14

Data Analysis: Descriptive and Inferential Statistics

INTRODUCTION

Measurement is critical to any study. The practitioner is interested in the similarity between the measurements used in a study and those usually found in his or her practice. The researcher thinks about how to measure relevant variables while reading the literature and thinking through the theoretical rationale for the study. Both the practitioner and the researcher wonder about how much faith they can put in the measurements reported.

Practitioners and researchers know that the perfect set of measurements does not exist. The researcher's task is to clearly define the variables, choose accurate measurement tools, and clearly explain how the statistical tools were used. Your task as a practitioner who critically reads research is to consider the researcher's explanation of how and why specific descriptive and inferential statistics were used and ask, "What do these numbers tell me?"

Descriptive statistics are valuable for summarizing data and allowing us to look at salient features about a group of data, but practitioners usually want more information. They want to be able to read about an intervention used with a specific group of individuals and consider the usefulness of that intervention with the patients in their care. The use of inferential statistics provides a way for practitioners to look at the data in a study and decide how easily the results can be generalized to the patients they see on a daily basis.

Initially, numbers tend to be intimidating. The best way to eliminate this source of intimidation is to jump in and play with the numbers. Keep reminding yourself that you have the intelligence and skills to do this. Use the mantras of "I think I can, I think I can" *(The Little Engine that Could)* and "practice, practice, practice," and you will have data analysis mastered. Also keep in mind that this is a life-long learning process. There will still be times when you will read a study with a new twist to the use of a statistical procedure, and back you'll go to the reference books, or pick up the phone to call a colleague.

This chapter is designed to help you with the skills part of the task. First, the exercises in this chapter will provide you with some practice in working with the concept of measurement. Second, you will have the opportunity to think through some of the decisions relevant to the use of descriptive and inferential statistics. The bulk of your effort will be spent digesting data from the studies included in the text.

LEARNING OUTCOMES

On completion of this chapter, the student should be able to do the following:

- Differentiate between descriptive and inferential statistics.
- State the purposes of descriptive statistics.

- Identify the levels of measurement in a research study.
- Describe a frequency distribution.
- List measures of central tendency and their use.
- List measures of variability and their use.
- Identify the purpose of inferential statistics.
- Explain the concept of probability as it applies to the analysis of sample data.
- Distinguish between a type I and type II error and its effect on a study's outcome.
- Distinguish between parametric and nonparametric tests.
- List some commonly used statistical tests and their purposes.
- Critically appraise the statistics used in published research studies.
- Evaluate the strength and quality of the evidence provided by the findings of a research study and determine their applicability to practice.

Activity 1

Before you start any of the activities for Chapter 14, make life easier for yourself—create tools that will provide a shortcut. Create a set of reference cards that can also serve as flash cards.

Create your own set of "statistical assistants." Once the cards are finished, carry them with you to the library, or set them on the desk while working on the Internet. Use them when reading research reports. Before long, you will be able to read a piece of research without referring to the stack of statistical assistants, and you will master the best shortcut of all: memorizing the statistical notation. Flipping through the pages of a book looking for a statistical symbol before you can evaluate the use of the statistic will no longer be required.

Gather the following supplies: package of 3 x 5 index cards, preferably lined on one side; pens or a combination of pens and highlighters with different colors; 1 broad-tipped, black-ink marker.

1. Make three key cards first. On one of the 3 x 5 cards, on the side without lines, use the broad-tipped, black marker and write "INFERENTIAL STATISTICAL TECHNIQUES—relationship" and on the second card write "INFERENTIAL STATISTICAL TECHNIQUES—difference." Take the third 3 x 5 card and write "DESCRIPTIVE TECHNIQUES" on the unlined side.

2. Turn the *inferential statistics—relationship* card over to the lined side. With one of the colored pens, write on the left side of the card the following list:

   two variables; interval measure
   two variables—nominal or ordinal
   >2 variables—interval measure
   >2 variables—nominal or ordinal

   Next to the descriptors at the left write the tests used for each type of data.

3. Turn the *inferential statistics—difference* card over to the lined side. With one of the colored pens, write on the left side of the card the following list:

   two groups—interval measure
   two groups—nominal or ordinal
   one group—interval measure
   one group—nominal or ordinal

   Next to the descriptors at the left write the tests used for each type of data.

4. Do the same with the *descriptive statistics* card. Write on the left side of the card the following list:

   nominal measurement
   ordinal measurement
   interval measurement
   ratio measurement

   Next to the descriptors at the left write the tests used for each type of data.

5. Each line of the key card should be in a different color. Next, create a stack of statistical assistants.

6. Take a blank card. On the front of each card (unlined side) write the full name of one of the statistical tools using the broad-tipped, black marker (or whatever marker was used to write on the front of the key card) (example: *mean*).

7. Turn the card over and write the information that corresponds to the appropriate category on the key card on the appropriate line using the appropriate color. If assistance with choosing the appropriate information to put on each line is needed, refer to Table 14-1, the descriptions of each test, in your textbook, and the Critical Thinking Decision Pathways in Chapter 14 of the text. For example, the lined side of the "mean" would read as follows:

   mathematical average of all scores
   interval or ratio data
   most used measure of central tendency, often used in tests of significance
   affected by every score, extreme scores can lead to big changes
   symbol: (see text)
   best point for summarizing interval or ratio data

8. These cards will fit into an envelope or any of the small plastic cases that can be purchased from the local bookstore. They will slip into a book bag, briefcase, or backpack with ease.

Activity 2

Match the level of measurement found in Column B with the appropriate example(s) in Column A. The levels of measurement in Column B will be used more than once. Table 14-1 from the text can assist you.

Column A

1. _____ Amount of emesis
2. _____ Scores on the ACT, SAT, or the GRE
3. _____ Height or weight
4. _____ High, moderate, low level of social support
5. _____ Satisfaction with nursing care
6. _____ Use or nonuse of contraception
7. _____ Class ranking
8. _____ Number of feet or meters walked
9. _____ Type A or type B behavior
10. _____ Body temperature measured with centi-grade thermometer

Column B

a. Nominal
b. Ordinal
c. Interval
d. Ratio

Activity 3

If you have taken a course in statistics, you are familiar with the statistical notation used to refer to specific types of descriptive statistics. This activity will serve as a quick review. If you have not yet taken a statistics course, this exercise will provide you with enough information to recognize some of the statistical notations.

This is a *reverse* crossword puzzle; therefore, the puzzle is already completed. Your task is to identify the appropriate clue for each answer found in the puzzle. List the correct clue answers in the spaces provided following the puzzle and clues.

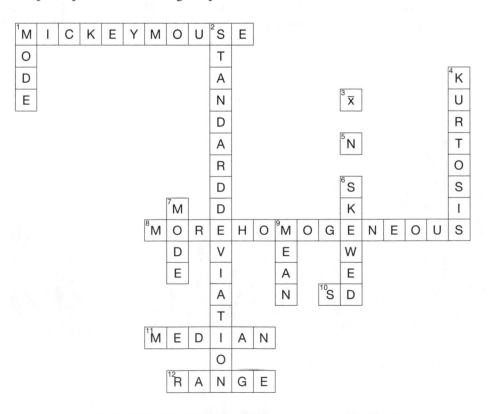

The Clues

a. Measure of central tendency used with interval or ratio data
b. Abbreviation for the number of measures in a given data set (the measures may be individual people or some smaller piece of data like blood pressure readings)
c. Measure of variation that shows the lowest and highest number in a set
d. Can describe the height of a distribution
e. Old abbreviation for the mean
f. Marks the "score" where 50% of the scores are higher and 50% are lower
g. Describes a distribution characterized by a tail
h. Abbreviation for standard deviation
i. 68% of the values in a normal distribution fall between +1 or –1 of this statistic
j. Goofy's best friend
k. Very unstable
l. The values that occur most frequently in a data set
m. Describes a set of data with a standard deviation of 3 when compared to a set of data with a standard deviation of 12

Across	Down
1.	1.
3.	2.
5.	4.
8.	6.
10.	7.
11.	9.
12.	

Activity 4

Read the following excerpts from specific studies. Identify both the independent and dependent variable(s) and indicate what level of measurement would apply. You may find the Critical Thinking Decision Path in the textbook to be very helpful in answering these questions.

1. "Participants were also asked to indicate how long they had experienced pain in their most painful location. Responses were coded into <1, 1–5, 6–10, 11–15 years, or more than15 years" (Horgas et al., 2008).

   a. Name the variable of interest.

   b. Identify the level of measurement of this variable.

2. "The hypothesis was supported. The mean total SRAHP score for the total sample ($n = 84$) was 77.87 (range 38–107, SD = 17.85) at time 1. SRAHP scores of total and of each subscale at time 1 were significantly higher in the comparison group ($p < .05$) than in the intervention group. Therefore, ANCOVA was used to test the effectiveness of the DHHI controlling

for self-efficacy score at time 1. Assumptions of ANCOVA were met. Total self-efficacy scores were significantly higher in the intervention group than in the comparison group after the DHHI, controlling for the total self-efficacy score at baseline (F [1,81]) = 26.02, $p < .05$)" (Jones et al., 2007).

    a. Name the independent variable(s).

    b. Name the dependent variable(s).

    c. Identify the level of measurement of the dependent variable.

3. "Pain. Chi-square analysis and t tests were conducted to examine the association between the presence of pain and race (Black or White); no statistically significant association was found ($\chi^2 = 2.32$, $df = 1$, $p = .09$). Blacks and Whites did not differ significantly in intensity ($t = -1.14$, $df = 44$, $p = .26$) or duration of self-reported pain ($\chi^2 = 3.68$, $df = 3$, $p = .30$), or in the number of pain locations reported ($t = -1.12$, $df = 67$, $p = .23$; see Table 2)" (Horgas et al., 2008).

    a. Name the variable(s).

    b. What level of measurement does a researcher need in order to use a chi-square test? What does this test measure?

Activity 5

Use the list of terms to complete the items in this activity. Some terms may be used more than once.

ANOVA	Correlation	Nonparametric statistics
Null hypothesis	Parameter	Parametric statistics
Practical significance	Probability	Research hypothesis
Sampling error	Statistic	Statistical significance
Type I error	Type II error	

1. The _____ states that there is no difference between the groups in the study or no association between the variables under study. Its usefulness to a study is that it is the only relationship that can be tested through the use of statistical tools.

2. ANOVA is an example of the use of _____.

3. It is impossible to prove that the _____ is true.

4. The tendency for statistics to fluctuate from one sample to another is known as the _____.

5. The term _____ refers to a characteristic of the population whereas the term _____ refers to a characteristic of a sample drawn from a population.

6. When investigators are studying the association between variables, they often will use statistics that measure _____.

7. _____ occurs when the investigator does not find statistical significance but a real difference exists in the world. A _____ occurs when the investigator concludes that there is a real (statistically significant) difference but, in reality, there is no difference.

8. The relative frequency of an event in repeated trials under similar conditions is known as _____ and provides the theoretical basis for inferential statistics.

9. A statistically significant finding based on a change of 3 mm Hg in systolic blood pressure in a sample of healthy individuals likely would have little _____.

10. _____ refer to those tools used when data are collected at the ordinal or nominal level of measurement.

11. When a finding is tested and found to be unlikely to have happened by chance, the investigators report _____ for that particular finding.

12. When a probability level is calculated as $p < 0.05$ and the investigator had set the alpha level of significance at 0.05, the investigator must reject the _____ and accept the _____.

13. Identify the components of the following statistical test result: χ^2 (6, $n = 213$) = 33.0, $p < .0001$. Match the component with its correct name.

_____	χ^2	a.	Sample size
_____	6	b.	Degrees of freedom
_____	$n = 213$	c.	Chi-square symbol
_____	33.0	d.	Probability level
_____	$p < .0001$	e.	Chi-square test statistic

Activity 6

The data in this table contains information from a study. Use the statistical assistant cards you developed in Activity 1 to answer the questions that follow Table 14-1.

Table 14-1: Demographic Data ($n = 12$) from Landreneau & Ward-Smith (2007)

Participant	Age	Gender	Marital Status	Ethnicity	Education	Income	Medical Status	Years in ESRD
#1	21	Female	Missing	Caucasian	10	Missing	Hypertension	5
#2	51	Female	Married	Caucasian	12	$10,001	Hypertension	2
#3	50	Male	Divorced	Caucasian	12	$60,001+	Diabetes mellitus Hypertension	1
#4	40	Male	Single	African American	BA	0+	Hypertension	2
#5	32	Female	Single	African American	12	0+	Hypertension	5
#6	77	Male	Married	Caucasian	MS	$30,001+	Diabetes mellitus Hypertension	1
#7	55	Male	Single	African American	6	0+	Hypertension	2
#8	44	Female	Married	Caucasian	GED	$10,001	Hypertension	2
#9	66	Male	Married	African American	12	0+	Diabetes mellitus Hypertension	2
#10	63	Female	Married	Caucasian	12	$10,001+	Hypertension	4
#11	Missing	Male	Missing	Missing	Missing	Missing	Missing	Missing
#12	58	Male	Single	African American	8	Missing	Diabetes mellitus Hypertension	4

Source: Landreneau KJ, Ward-Smith P: Perceptions of adult patients on hemodialysis concerning choice among renal replacement therapies, *Nephrol Nurs* 34(5):513-519, 525, 2007.

1. How big is the sample size?

2. What levels of measurement are represented by the data in this table?

3. For the data in the last column, Years in ESRD, what is the mean?

4. For the data in the last column, Years in ESRD, what is the median?

5. For the data in the last column, Years in ESRD, what is the mode?

6. What is a limitation of using the mean to describe this sample?

Activity 7

Using the studies in Appendices A through D in the textbook, answer the following questions regarding the use of descriptive and inferential statistics in each study. Once again, use the Critical Thinking Decision Path in Chapter 14 of the textbook.

1. Were descriptive statistics used in the study?

   a. Meneses et al.

   b. Jones et al.

   c. Horgas et al.

   d. Landreneau et al.

2. What data were summarized and/or explained through the use of descriptive statistics?

   a. Meneses et al.

   b. Jones et al.

   c. Horgas et al.

   d. Landreneau et al.

3. Were the descriptive statistics used appropriately?

   a. Meneses et al.

   b. Jones et al.

   c. Horgas et al.

   d. Landreneau et al.

4. Did any of the four studies rely more heavily on the use of descriptive statistics than the others? If so, why do you think this occurred?

5. Now turn to the inferential statistics. Which of the four studies in the appendices used some type of inferential statistic to manage the data?

   a. Meneses et al.

   b. Jones et al.

   c. Horgas et al.

   d. Landreneau et al.

6. Name the inferential statistical tools used in the studies.

   a. Meneses et al.

   b. Jones et al.

   c. Horgas et al.

   d. Landreneau et al.

Activity 8: Web-Based Activity

Go to www.cdc.gov and click on "Injury, Violence, and Safety" on the middle of the Web page. Click on the "Teen Driver Safety" site. Scroll down and skim the contents of this site.

1. How much more likely are teen drivers to crash than older drivers? What are some factors that increase this risk?

2. What percent of teen deaths from motor vehicle crashes occur on Friday, Saturday, or Sunday?

Activity 9: Evidence-Based Practice Activity

Evidence-based practice means that you base practice decisions on the best evidence available. In the ideal world, this means practitioners would have a stack of experimental studies with clear conclusions that have direct relevance to an immediate clinical concern. Obviously, this is seldom the case. We use our brains and the best practice information available, and intervene and evaluate.

Assume that the CDC statistics from Activity 8 about teen drivers have been consistently reported across several studies of varying designs and sample sizes. What, if any, implications would exist for RNs working as school nurses in high schools?

POSTTEST

1. Two outpatient clinics measured client waiting time as one indicator of effectiveness. The mean and standard deviation of waiting time in minutes is reported below. Which outpatient clinic would you prefer, assuming that all other things are equal? Explain your answer.

	Clinic 1	Clinic 2
Mean (in minutes)	40	25
Standard deviation (in minutes)	10	45

2. You are responsible for ordering a new supply of hospital gowns for your unit. Which measure of central tendency would be the most useful in your decision making? Explain your answer.

REFERENCES

Horgas AL, Yoon S, Nichols AL, et al.: The relationship between pain and functional disability in black and white older adults, *Res Nurs Health* 31:1-14, 2008.

Jones EG, Renger R, Kang Y: Self-efficacy for health related behaviors among deaf adults, *Res Nurs Health* 30:185-192, 2007.

Landreneau KJ, Ward-Smith P: Perceptions of adult patients on hemodialysis concerning choice among renal replacement therapies, *Nephrol Nurs* 34(5):513-519, 525, 2007.

Meneses KD, McNees P, Loerzel VW, et al.: Transition from treatment to survivorship: Effects of a psychoeducational intervention on quality of life in breast cancer survivors, *Oncol Nurs Forum* 34(5):1007-1016, 2007.

U.S. Department of Health and Human Services: Centers for Disease Control. Retrieved August 28, 2009, from www.cdc.gov.

15

Understanding Research Findings

INTRODUCTION

As the last sections of a research report, the results and conclusions sections answer the question "So what?" In other words, it is in these two sections that the investigator "makes sense" of the research, critically synthesizes the data, ties them to a theoretical framework, and builds on a body of knowledge. These two sections are a very important part of the research report because they describe the generalizability of the findings and offer recommendations for further research. Well-written, clear, and concise results and conclusions sections provide valuable information for nursing practice. Conversely, poorly written results and conclusions sections will leave a reader bewildered, confused, and wondering how or if the findings are relevant to nursing.

LEARNING OUTCOMES

On completion of this chapter, the student should be able to do the following:

- Discuss the difference between the "Results" and the "Discussion of the Results" sections of a research article.
- Identify the format and components of the "Results" section.
- Determine if both statistically supported and statistically unsupported findings are appropriately discussed.
- Determine whether the results are objectively reported.
- Describe how tables and figures are used in a research report.
- List the criteria of a meaningful table.
- Identify the format and components of the "Discussion" section.
- Determine the purpose of the "Discussion" section.
- Discuss the importance of including generalizability and limitations of a study in the report.
- Determine the purpose of including recommendations in the study report.
- Discuss how the strength, quality, and consistency of evidence provided by the findings are related to a study's results, limitations, generalizability, and applicability to practice.

Activity 1

Knowing what information to look for and where to find it in the "Results" and "Discussions" sections of a research report will enable you to interpret the research findings and critique research reports.

Identify the section in which the following information from the research report may be found. Put an **R** in the blank space if the information would be found in the "Results" section and a **D** if the information would be found in the "Discussion" section.

1. _____ Tables/figures

2. _____ Limitations of the study

3. _____ Data analysis related to the literature review

4. _____ Inferences or generalization of results

5. _____ Statistical support or nonsupport of hypotheses

6. _____ Findings of the hypothesis testing

7. _____ Information about the statistical tests used to analyze hypotheses

8. _____ Application of meaning (makes sense) of data analysis

9. _____ Suggestions for further research

10. _____ Recommendations for nursing practice

Activity 2

Tables are an important part of the data analysis component of a study. This activity will focus on tables.

Read the following paragraph from the Jones et al. (2007) study on self-efficacy for health behaviors in deaf adults. Then review the data in Table 1 from the same study (on the next page). Answer the questions that follow the table.

"A sample of 105 deaf adults was recruited in Phoenix and Tucson, Arizona. The 84 participants who completed both time-1 and time-2 data collection included more women (58%) than men, and had a median education level of high school and a mean age of 51 years (range 18–85, SD = 18.34). There was a significant difference between the intervention and comparison groups in ethnic composition (composition $\chi^2[1, N = 84] = 8.17, p = .004$), with more participants in the intervention group (37%) who were members of ethnic minorities (mainly Mexican-American) than in the comparison group (8%)" (Jones et al., 2007).

Table 15-1: Demographic Characteristics of Participants in Jones et al. (2007)

Variable	Intervention Group ($n = 32$)	Comparison Group ($n = 52$)
Age		
M ± SD (range)	51.3 ± 15.4 (18 – 83)	50.6 ± 20.1 (22 – 85)
Education		
M ± SD (range)	11.8 ± 2.9 (5 – 8)	11.9 ± 3.5 (4 – 20)
Sex		
Men	14 (43.8%)	21 (40.4 %)
Women	18 (57.2%)	31 (59.6%)
Ethnicity		
White (NH*)	20 (62.5%)	45 (86.4%)
Hispanic (MA**)	10 (31.3%)	2 (3.8%)
African American	0 (0.0%)	2 (3.8%)
Other	2 (6.2%)	2 (3.8%)
Missing	0	1 (2.1%)
Living Situation		
Married/partnered	15 (46.9%)	17 (32.7%)
Single	16 (50.0%)	34 (65.4%)
Missing	1 (3.1%)	1 (1.9%)

Source: Jones EG, Renger R, Kang Y: Self-efficacy for health-related behaviors among deaf adults, *Res Nurs Health* 30:185-192, 2007.

1. Does the information in the table meet the criteria for a table as described in Chapter 15 of the textbook? Explain.

2. What was the most common ethnicity?

3. Were more participants married or single?

4. What information is presented in the text but cannot be found in the table?

Activity 3

Collect demographic data on the people in your research class. You can decide what data you want to collect, but common variables would be age, gender, eye color, hair color (current or underlying), and so on. Once the data have been collected, work in groups of no fewer than three but no more than five and create a table that displays these data. Exchange tables with another group. Critique each other's table with the intent of improving the table.

Criteria to consider:

a. Are data summaries included and not all of the raw data?
b. Is the title clear? Do you know what data are being presented without needing to read the text?
c. Are the columns and rows appropriately labeled?
d. Are there other criteria you want to include? Does your instructor have suggestions?

Activity 4

This activity will give you some practice in the interpretation of research articles. Read the Meneses et al. (2007) article in Appendix A of the textbook and answer the following items.

1. The following items pertain to Table 1 of the article.

   a. What is the meaning of the "(experimental group $N = 125$)" on this table?

   b. Where was the standard deviation largest? What does SD measure?

   c. What data did you use to answer item b? Based on these data, where would you expect to find 68% of the scores for this group?

   d. What does a p value of 0.001 mean?

2. The following data are extracted from Table 2 in Meneses et al. (2007):

Covariate Adjustment	Without Covariates	p
Overall quality of life	-4.356	<0.001
Physical well-being	-1.129	0.258
Psychological well-being	-4.994	<0.001
Social well-being	-2.974	0.003
Spiritual well-being	-0.704	40.482

   a. Which results are statistically significant ($p < 0.001$)?

   b. Do you agree with the authors' conclusions on why the intervention was effective in the psychological domain but less effective for physical well-being? (Hint: Reread the "Discussion" section.)

Activity 5: Web-Based Activity

1. Go to your library Web page and open your favorite database. Now type "analysis research studies, nursing" in the search box. How many hits did you get? Skim through the first five pages of listed items. What words seem to be driving the search?

2. Now add the term "statistical analysis" to your previous search. If you get too many results, try to find articles with this phrase in the title. How many studies did you pull up? Read the first study and see what statistical analysis was performed on a nursing research problem. What was the analysis?

Activity 6: Evidence-Based Practice Activity

Evidence-based practice asks the practitioner to use the "best" evidence available when deciding which interventions to use. The results and discussion section of any study can help you, the knowledgeable consumer of research, decide if the study is one that needs to be included in your considerations.

Go to your library Web page and click on a nursing journal you like or have used previously. Is the journal peer reviewed? If you were looking at a research study in your field with potential impact on your practice, would you consider peer review as part of your critique process? What are the specific instructions for authors? How are statistical results and results in general reported?

POSTTEST

1. When a research hypothesis is supported through testing, it may be assumed that the hypothesis was which of the following?
   a. Proved
   b. Accepted
   c. Rejected
   d. Disconfirmed

2. Limitations of a study describe its weaknesses.

   True   False

3. The "Results" section of a research study includes all the following *except:*
   a. Hypothesis testing results
   b. Tables and figures
   c. Statistical test description
   d. Limitations of the study

4. Unsupported hypotheses mean that the study is of little value in improving practice.

   True   False

5. Tables in research reports should meet all of the following criteria *except:*
   a. Clear and concise
   b. Restate the text narrative
   c. Economize the text
   d. Supplement the text narrative

6. The "Discussion" section provides opportunity for the investigator to do all of the following *except:*
   a. Describe implications from the research results
   b. Relate the results to the literature review
   c. Make generalizations to large populations of subjects
   d. Suggest areas for further research

7. Hypothesis testing is described in the "Discussion" section of the research report.

   True   False

REFERENCES

Jones EG, Renger R, Kang Y: Self-efficacy for health-related behaviors among deaf adults, *Res Nurs Health* 30:185-192, 2007.

Meneses DK, McNees P, Loerzel W, et al.: Transition from treatment to survivorship: Effects of a psychoeducational intervention on quality of life in breast cancer survivors, *Oncol Nurs Forum* 34:1007-1016, 2007.

16

Appraising Quantitative Research

INTRODUCTION

Chapter 16 in the textbook includes two thorough critiques of two quantitative studies. The first study critiqued is a study by Massey (2007) that evaluated the effect of rocking-chair motion on postoperative ileus in abdominal surgery patients. The second critique is on a study by Howell et al. (2007) that examined relationships among anxiety, anger, and blood pressure in elementary school–age children. Critiquing criteria that have been presented in all previous chapters are combined and utilized. The result is a complete critique of two separate studies.

Both of these critiques reflect the level of analysis desired for an article that the RN had decided was relevant to practice. If you want to produce a critique at this level of thoroughness, it will take time. It would not be uncommon for a novice reader of research to use 2 to 3 hours (maybe more) to complete such a critique. Usually, novice readers of research find the task tedious and, not infrequently, difficult. The more often you read and critique studies in this manner, the easier (and more interesting) reading research becomes. The easier it becomes, the more quickly you can complete a critique. To get started, you just have to pick an article, dive in, and do it.

One way of getting started is to work on a weekly schedule to master this skill. Each week, find one research article relevant to an area of nursing you are interested in and critique that article using the steps outlined in the textbook. At the end of 1 year, you will have read four dozen studies (take time off for holidays, your birthday, and one "I just forgot"). By this time, you will have mastered research critiques.

As mentioned earlier, this level of reading and critiquing is most often used when you have a reasonable expectation that a specific study will be useful in your professional practice. But not all relevant articles will be found in the journals that are devoted specifically to your area of clinical expertise. You must search several journals to find all of the articles that can be useful. When you do find an article that appears to be practice-relevant, you need to assess the article quickly so you can decide whether it requires more in-depth analysis.

LEARNING OUTCOMES

On completion of this chapter, the student should be able to do the following:

- Identify the purpose of the critical appraisal process.
- Describe the criteria for each step of the critical appraisal process.
- Describe the strengths and weaknesses of a research report.
- Assess the strength, quality, and consistency of evidence provided by a quantitative research report.

- Discuss applicability of the findings of a research report for evidence-based nursing practice.
- Conduct a critique of a research report.

Activity 1

This quick reading of articles demands that you, the reader, consider the same aspects of a study that you would consider if completing a more detailed critique but in a more superficial manner. This type of reading is called "inspectional reading" (Adler & Van Doren, 1972). Mastering inspectional reading is essential, but is frequently overlooked in regard to analytical skills. Frequently, professional reading must be squeezed into a small window of available time. Improving your quick reading skills will help you to sort through the reading that is required to maintain and expand your knowledge base.

But what is this inspectional reading? It is the second level in a set of skills described by Adler and Van Doren (1972). The first skill is elementary reading, which is usually accomplished by the time you have completed the fourth grade. Level two is inspectional reading. Level three is analytical reading where the reader is trying very hard to understand what the author is attempting to share, and is the level of reading required to produce a critique of a research study. Level four is syntopical reading, which requires intense effort to synthesize ideas from many sources.

Inspectional reading has two components. The first is called "systematic skimming" and the second is called "superficial reading."

Systematic skimming is the first thing anyone should do when approaching a reading assignment. It requires only a few minutes to skim an article (it may take up to an hour if you are skimming a complete book). Let's assume that you are going to skim a hard copy of a research article.

- Read the title and the abstract.
- Read the biographical information about the authors/researchers.
- Pay close attention to the clinical area and the population of subjects.
- Read the conclusions section.
- Ask yourself the following questions: "Are the individuals in this study comparable to the people I am interested in? Is the problem/clinical area/question close to my interests?" If you answer "no" to these questions, put this study down and go to the next one. If you answer "yes" to either of these questions, proceed to superficial reading of the article.

If you are undecided about whether it is related to your clinical concerns, proceed to superficial reading of the article.

Superficial reading requires that you read the article from beginning to end without stopping. Do not take notes. Do not highlight. (Hide your highlighter so you won't even be tempted.) Do not use the dictionary to understand words that you don't know. Do not stop and think "I wonder what they meant by that." Just read!

When you have completed the article, take a deep breath and ask yourself these questions:

- What do I remember about the study? The question? The methods? The results? The discussion?
- Was this clinical or basic research?
- Was it experimental, nonexperimental, or qualitative?
- Where would I put it on the level of evidence scale?
- Did anything in the study raise any ethical questions? (Listen to yourself. If there is even a twinge of a question, listen to yourself.)

- Does it fit my interests? (If the answer is "no," move on to the next article. If the answer is "maybe," put it in a come-back-to-later stack. If the answer is "yes," proceed to more detailed reading and perhaps jot down the notes that would be necessary to complete a critique.)

Now let's practice. There is one activity for this chapter. The Meneses et al. (2007) article (Appendix A of the textbook) has been used for several activities throughout this study guide. However, it is possible that you have not read it completely from beginning to end. **Do so now.** Read the Meneses et al. (2007) article using the inspectional reading strategies. When you have completed reading the article, answer the questions related to inspectional reading. Make a decision: Is this an article that would assist you in building the evidence base for the area of nursing that most appeals to you?

When you have completed your reading, turn to the answers in the back of the study guide. *Note:* There is no posttest for this chapter. Enjoy the break!

REFERENCES

Adler MJ, Van Doren C: *How to read a book,* New York, 1972, Simon & Schuster.

Meneses DK, McNees P, Loerzel W, et al.: Transition from treatment to survivorship: Effects of a psychoeducational intervention on quality of life in breast cancer survivors, *Oncol Nurs Forum* 34:1007-1016, 2007.

Developing an Evidence-Based Practice

INTRODUCTION

Engaging in evidence-based practice has become an expected standard in the delivery of health care services. Although there are concentrated efforts on methods to facilitate the translation of research findings into practice, nurses can engage in evidence-based practice through the development, implementation, and evaluation of evidence-based practice guidelines that can improve patient outcomes. This chapter pulls together many of the Evidence-Based Practice Tips that have been included in the previous chapters to provide you with strategies to develop your own evidence-based nursing practice.

LEARNING OUTCOMES

On completion of this chapter, the student should be able to do the following:

- Differentiate among conduct of nursing research, research utilization, and evidence-based practice.
- Describe the steps of evidence-based practice.
- Identify three barriers to evidence-based practice and strategies to address each.
- List three sources for finding evidence.
- Describe strategies for implementing evidence-based practice changes.
- Identify steps for evaluating an evidence-based change in practice.
- Use research findings and other forms of evidence to improve the quality of care.

Activity 1

Although the terms *research utilization* and *evidence-based practice* are often used interchangeably, they are not "one and the same" (Titler et al., 1999). Answer the following to help you differentiate between the two terms.

1. Describe the difference between *research utilization* and *evidence-based practice*.

2. Identify the three major components of *evidence-based practice.*

a. _____

b. _____

c. _____

Activity 2

Following are short descriptions of RN activities related to research. Each can be categorized as one of the following:

A. Conduct of research
B. Dissemination of research findings
C. Research utilization
D. Evidence-based practice

Place the letter (A, B, C, D) that best describes each activity in the space provided.

1. _____   The RN submits an article to his or her health care agency's in-house practice newsletter about the research study he or she participated in.

2. _____   As a member of the health care team, the RN was involved with developing a plan of care for a patient using the findings from one meta-analysis and several research studies.

3. _____   Two RNs are involved with data collection for a study comparing two types of dressings for postoperative incisions.

4. _____   The RN has read about an intervention that will reduce the pain associated with the injection of a particular medication. After reviewing all of the variables, he or she decides that trying the intervention would be a good idea and proceeds to develop an implementation plan.

5. _____   Marie has been working with a faculty member on an independent study project. The two of them have decided to publish the results of their work.

6. _____   A journal club group comprised of RNs, MDs, and NPs have identified specific clinical question and plan to develop a practice guideline by the end of the year.

Activity 3

Number the following major steps of evidence-based practice in the correct sequence. Use the number "1" for the first step.

a. _____   Choose a systematic approach for grading the evidence (the quality of the individual evidence and strength of the body of evidence)

b. _____   Select a topic

c. _____   Critique research evidence (systematic reviews including meta-analyses and/or meta-syntheses; primary sources/individual research studies)

d. _____   Implement the evidence-based practice change

e. _____   Form a team

f. _____   Evaluate the evidence-based practice change

g. _____   Critique existing evidence-based practice guidelines

h. _____   Identify evidence-based practice change recommendations

i. _____   Develop/write the evidence-based practice change in detail

j. _____   Retrieve the best-available evidence

k. _____   Synthesize the evidence

l. _____   Identify stakeholders

m. _____   Identify a method for evaluating the effectiveness of the evidence-based practice change

n. _____   Decide if a change in practice is warranted

Activity 4

Fill in the blanks with the appropriate word(s) from the text.

1. There are two forms of using research evidence in practice. _____-driven evidence influences thinking, whereas _____-driven evidence endorses current practice or practice change.

2. Clinical questions arise from different types of "triggers." _____ triggers occur when staff members interact directly with patients or with direct care-related situations, whereas _____ triggers are generated during activities such as reviewing existing evidence-based practice guidelines or attending conferences where research findings are being disseminated.

3. Formulating clinical questions is the key to retrieving the best-available evidence for an identified topic. PICO is one such effective approach to formulating clinical questions. Identify the four components of this acronym: P _____; I _____; C _____; O _____

4. A team is responsible for the development, implementation, and evaluation of an evidence-based practice project. This team is likely to include _____, who are key individuals who will be affected by the implementation of evidence-based practice project and who are critical to its successful implementation.

Activity 5: Web-Based Activity

As evidence-based practice guidelines become increasingly important, it is crucial that clinicians be able to critique these guidelines with regard to the methods used in developing them and considering the use of existing guidelines in practice. In addition, critique of existing guidelines provides clinicians with a sense of how evidence-based practice guidelines should be developed.

Retrieve the AGREE tool for critiquing guidelines from www.agreecollaboration.org and critique the guideline titled "Prevention and Management of Dental Decay in the Pre-school Child" (Uribe, 2006). Critique the guideline by Uribe using the AGREE tool. Answers will be provided in the Study Guide Answer Key. After you complete the critical appraisal using the AGREE tool, search for this guideline on the National Guideline Clearinghouse (www.guideline.gov). Compare your critical appraisal using the AGREE tool to the information you retrieve from the National Guideline Clearinghouse.

Activity 6

A critical step in evidence-based practice is to retrieve evidence, such as evidence-based practice guidelines (Level I Evidence). Identify five sources (along with their websites) where you would begin your search for the best-available evidence-based practice guidelines.

a. _____

b. _____

c. _____

d. _____

Activity 7

Once evidence-base practice recommendations have been developed from the critique and synthesis of the best-available evidence, it is then important to determine if these recommendations should result in a evidence-based practice change. Indicate *yes (Y)* or *no (N)* as to whether the following should be considered in making this decision. The extent to which:

1. _____ there are similar findings reported using different study designs.

2. _____ the evidence was published in peer-reviewed journals.

3 _____ the sample characteristics in the study designs are representative of the target population (population in which the evidence-based practice change is going to be implemented).

4. _____ the studies support current practice.

5. _____ the authors of the studies and/or guidelines are well-known in their field.

6. _____ there are similar findings reported using similar study designs.

Activity 8

Although a practice change may be evidence-based, its adoption depends on several factors. The answers the following questions will help to identify factors influencing the adoption of an evidence-based practice change.

1. There are several organization factors that affect the adoption of evidence-based practice changes. Which of the following is considered in your text to be the most important organizational factor?

   a. organizational size
   b. leadership support
   c. absorptive capacity
   d. organizational culture

2. In order to address such organizational factors, interventions to improve the implementation and adoption of evidence-based practice changes are discussed in terms of five major categories. Identify these categories.

   a. _____

   b. _____

   c. _____

   d. _____

   e. _____

3. There are several strategies to promote the adoption related to the characteristics of evidence-based practice changes. Which of the following significantly improves adoption on the basis of the characteristics of an evidence-based practice change?
   a. How important the evidence-based practice change is to stakeholders
   b. The use of practitioner review and "reinvention"
   c. The use of computer knowledge management
   d. How easy the evidence-based practice change is to implement

4. Education is necessary for practice change. Which one of the following has shown positive effects on improving the adoption of evidence-based practice change?
   a. interactive education
   b. interprofessional education
   c. discipline-specific education
   d. didactic education

5. Using multiple methods of communication, such as mass media, consultation with experts, and education, is a strategy that has been used to promote evidence-based practice change. List three additional strategies that are being used to promote such change.

   a. _____

   b. _____

   c. _____

Activity 9: Web-Based Activity

Retrieve and review the following:

Centre for Evidence-Based Healthcare, Evidence-Based Medicine Informatics Project: How to use clinical practice guidelines, 2001. Retrieved September 1, 2009, from www.cche.net/usersguides/guidelines.asp.
Graham ID, Harrison MB: Evaluation and adaptation of clinical practice guidelines, *Evidence-Based Nursing* 8:68-72, 2005.
Thomas L: Clinical practice guidelines, *Evidence-Based Nursing* 2:2, 1999.

POSTTEST

Retrieve the article by Poppleton, Moynihan, and Hickey (2003). Based on the article, answer the following questions about evidence-based practice change.

1. What was the overall topic of the evidence-based practice guideline(s)?

2. Who were members of the evidence-based practice guideline team?

3. Who, if anyone, would you identify as "stakeholders" in the evidence-based practice guideline team? Is there anyone not represented?

4. Was the best-available evidence retrieved? If so, which strategies were used?

5. What was the approach for grading the quality of the individual evidence and strength of the body of evidence?

6. Was the research evidence (existing clinical practice guidelines, systematic reviews [including meta-analyses and/or meta-syntheses], and primary sources/individual research studies) critiqued?

7. Was the research evidence synthesized? What were the evidence-based practice change recommendations?

8. Was the evidence-based practice change written in detail?

9. How was the decision to make the evidence-based practice change supported?

10. Is a method for evaluating the effectiveness of the evidence-based practice change identified?

11. Was the evidence-based practice change evaluated? Was it successful?

12. What were the strategies used by the evidence-based change team to promote the adoption of the evidence-based practice change?

REFERENCES

Centre for Evidence-Based Healthcare, Evidence-Based Medicine Informatics Project: How to use clinical practice guidelines, 2001. Retrieved September 1, 2009, from www.cche.net/usersguides/guideline.asp.

Graham ID, Harrison MB: Evaluation and adaptation of clinical practice guidelines, *Evidence-Based Nursing* 8:68-72, 2005.

Poppleton VK, Moynihan PJ, Hickey PA: Clinical practice guidelines: the Boston experience, *Prog Pediatr Cardiol* 18:75-83, 2003.

Thomas L: Clinical practice guidelines, *Evidence-Based Nursing* 2:2, 1999.

Titler MG, Mentes JC, Rakel BA, et al.: From book to bedside: Putting evidence to use in the care of the elderly, *Jt Comm J Qual Improv* 25(10):545-556, 1999.

Uribe S: Prevention and management of dental decay in the pre-school child, *Evidence-Based Dentistry* 7:1, 2006.

18

Tools for Applying Evidence to Practice

INTRODUCTION

The development of evidence-based nursing practice depends on applying new evidence to practice. This chapter provides you with tools that you need to ask clinical questions, search the literature for the best-available evidence, and appraise the best-available evidence according to category and design. Equipped with these tools, you will have knowledge to be able to arrive at clinical decisions based on the best-available evidence combined with clinical expertise and patient preferences.

LEARNING OUTCOMES

After reading this chapter, the student should be able to do the following:

- Identify the key elements of a focused clinical question.
- Discuss the use of databases to search the literature.
- Screen a research article for relevance and credibility.
- Critically appraise study results and apply the findings to individual patients.
- Make clinical decisions based on evidence from the literature combined with clinical expertise and patient preferences.

Activity 1

Using the PICO format to organize a clinical question is helpful to the nurse who is searching for the best-available evidence. In addition to determining major search terms, the PICO format also helps the nurse to determine the clinical category to which a research study belongs. Follow the instruction below:

(A) Put the following clinical questions into PICO format.

(B) Identify which of the clinical categories you would expect the study to belong to:

> *Therapy (T)*
> *Diagnosis (D)*
> *Prognosis(P)*
> *Causation/Harm (C/H)*

1. In older adults, do measures of adiposity and cardiorespiratory fitness predict mortality? (Peters, 2008)

   a. P _____

   _____

   b. I _____

   _____

   c. C _____

   _____

   d. O _____

   _____

   e. Clinical Category: _____

2. Is negative pressure wound therapy (NPWT) using vacuum-assisted closure more effective than advanced moist wound therapy (AMWT) for diabetic foot ulcers? (Sandison, 2008)

   a. P _____

   _____

   b. I _____

   _____

   c. C _____

   _____

   d. O _____

   _____

   e. Clinical Category: _____

3. What is the accuracy of the CRAFFT test in screening for substance abuse among adolescents in a hospital-based clinic? (Jull, 2003)

    a. P _____

       _____

    b. I _____

       _____

    c. C _____

       _____

    d. O _____

       _____

    e. Clinical Category: _____

4. Is there an association between the risk of childhood acute lymphoblastic leukemia and residential exposure to magnetic fields from power lines? (Bryant-Lukosius, 1998)

    a. P _____

       _____

    b. I _____

       _____

    c. C _____

       _____

    d. O _____

       _____

    e. Clinical Category: _____

Activity 2: Web-Based Activity

As mentioned above, determining the clinical category of a research study will help in your search for the best-available evidence. Access the following online bibliographic databases and list the clinical category filters for each database below.

1. CINAHL

2. MEDLINE

3. PUBMED (Medline)—click "Limits" on top of homepage

4. PUBMED (Medline)—click on "Clinical Queries" on left side of homepage

5. Based on the clinical category filters for each of the bibliographic databases above, which database do you think would provide you the most efficient search if you were able to identify the clinical category of the PICO question you were searching for?

Activity 3

As an RN working in a primary care clinic located in Miami, Florida, you are concerned with the number of adolescent type 2 diabetic patients who have difficulty maintaining a hemoglobin $A_{1C} < 7.0\%$. You perform a literature review to see if there are any interventions that the primary care clinic can use to help these patients. You retrieve the randomized control trial by Peterson et al. (2008). The following is a summary of the design and findings (Whittemore, 2009). Use this information to answer the questions below.

Setting: 24 family medicine/internal medicine primary care practices in Minnesota

Sample: $N = 8,405$ patients ages 18 to 89 years old

Methods: concealed, unblinded

Intervention: TRANSLATE intervention

Control: usual quality improvement

Findings: 49% of patients in the intervention group and 44% of patients in the control group achieved a hemoglobin $A_{1C} < 7.0\%$. The RBI (95% CI) was 12% (6 to 18) and the NNT (CI) was 20 (14 to 35).

1. What was the PICO question addressed in the clinical situation?

2. What is the PICO question addressed in the study by Peterson et al. (2008)?

3. How do the PICO questions in addressed in the clinical situation and in the study by Peterson et al. (2008) compare?

4. Did the patients know whether they had been assigned to the control or intervention group?

5. How was the outcome variable measured? Was it measured as a continuous or discrete variable?

6. What is the null value of the outcome measure used to interpret the CI?

7. Interpret the RBI and NNT.

8. Are the RBI and NNT statistically significant? (Hint: Consider the CIs.)

9. Is the NNT clinically significant?

10. How would you apply the results of this study to the clinical situation? Do the results warrant an evidence-based practice change?

Activity 4

You are volunteering with a school nurse at a local high school San Francisco, California. In your first few weeks of volunteering you start to wonder why it seems that most of the teenage girls being diagnosed with eating disorders are those whose parents are divorced. Out of curiosity, you perform a quick literature review to see if the evidence supports what your observations. You retrieve the cohort study by Martínez-González et al., (2003). The following is a summary of the design and findings (Newton, 2003). Use this information to answer the questions below:

Setting: Navarra, Spain

Sample: $N = 2,862$ girls ages 12 to 21 years old (mean age 15.5 years old)

Outcomes: parents' marital status (other versus married); eating alone (yes versus no); reading girls' magazines (< weekly versus ≥ weekly); and listening to radio (≤ 1 hour per day versus > 1 hour per day)

Findings: when odds ratios (CI 95%) were adjusted for all variables as well as age, body mass index, self-esteem, and socioeconomic status, of the girls who were clinically diagnoses with eating disorders ($n = 90$) findings indicated that the OR for parents' marital status was 1.97 (1.10 to 3.51), for eating alone was 2.94 (1.88 to 4.60), for reading girls' magazines was 1.42 (0.91 to 2.2), and for listening to radio was 1.55 (1.01 to 2.40).

1. What was the PICO question addressed in the clinical situation?

2. The question addressed in the study by Peterson et al. (2008) was, "Are parental, mass media, sociodemographic, and psychosocial variables associated with an increased risk of developing an eating disorder (ED) in girls?" (Newton, 2003, p. 120). How do the PICO questions in addressed in the clinical situation and in the study by Peterson et al. (2008) compare?

3. Based on the PICO question of the clinical situation and the question addressed in the study by Peterson et al. (2008), what clinical category is being addressed? Structured tools are available to help you systematically appraise the strength and quality of evidence for a given category of a clinical question. Although many tools exist, the tools developed by the Critical Appraisal Skills Programme (CASP) are easily accessible and user-friendly to complete. Go to the CASP website (www.phru.nhs.uk/pages/PHD/resources.htm) to determine which of the tools you use to critique the study by Peterson et al. (2008).

4. Indicate whether each of the outcomes are continuous variables (C) or discrete variables (D).

   a. _____ parents' marital status

   b. _____ eating alone

   c. _____ reading girls' magazines

   d. _____ listening to radio

5. Interpret the study findings. Which findings are statistically significant? How can you tell?

6. How would you apply the results of this study to the clinical situation? Do the results warrant an evidence-based practice change?

Activity 5: Web-Based Activity

Retrieve and review the following:

Bassler D, Busse JW, Karanicolas PJ, Guyatt GH: Evidence-based practice targets the individual patient. Part 1: how clinicians can use study results to determine optimal individual care, *Evidence-Based Nursing* 11:103-104, 2008.

Ciliska D, Cullum N, Marks S: Evaluation of systematic reviews for treatment or prevention interventions, *Evidence-Based Nursing* 4:100-104, 2001.

DiCenso A: Clinically useful measures of the effects of treatment, *Evidence-Based Nursing* 4:36-39, 2001.

POSTTEST

Determine whether each of the following statements is True (T) or False (F). If an item is False, revise it to make it a True statement.

1. _____ An experimental or quasi-experimental study design is usually used for the causation/harm category of clinical concern used by clinicians.

2. _____ Articles should be screened to determine if the setting and sample in the study are similar to my clinical situation.

3. _____ A confidence interval can provide the reader information about the statistical significance of the findings.

4. _____ Every systematic review is a meta-analysis.

5. _____ *Specificity* is the term used to describe the proportion of individuals with a disease who test positive for it.

6. _____ A confidence interval does not provide the reader information about the clinical significance of the findings.

7. _____ The null value for continuous variables is "0."

8. _____ *NNT* is a useful measure for applying research findings to practice.

9. _____ Every meta-analysis is a systematic review.

10. _____ *Prevalence* is a term used to describe the number that expresses the sensitivity, specificity, PPV, and NPV.

REFERENCES

Bassler D, Busse JW, Karanicolas PJ, Guyatt GH: Evidence-based practice targets the individual patient. Part 1: how clinicians can use study results to determine optimal individual care, *Evidence-Based Nursing* 11:103-104, 2008.

Bryant-Lukosius D (1998). Childhood acute lymphoblastic leukaemia was not linked to residential exposure to power line magnetic fields. *Evidence-Based Nursing*, 1, 55.

Ciliska D, Cullum N, Marks S: Evaluation of systematic reviews for treatment or prevention interventions, *Evidence-Based Nursing* 4:100-104, 2001.

DiCenso A: Clinically useful measures of the effects of treatment, *Evidence-Based Nursing* 4:36-39, 2001.

Jull A: The CRAFFT test was accurate for screening substance abuse among adolescent clinic patients, *Evidence-Based Nursing* 6:23, 2003.

Martínez-González MA, Gual P, Lahortiga F, et al.: Parental factors, mass media influences, and the onset of eating disorders in a prospective population-based cohort, *Pediatrics* 111:315-320, 2003.

Newton M: Eating alone, parents' marital status, and use of radio and girls' magazines were risk factors for eating disorders, *Evidence-Based Nursing* 6:120, 2003.

Peters A: BMI and cardiorespiratory fitness predicted mortality in older adults, *Evidence-Based Medicine* 13:90-91, 2008.

Peterson KA, Radosevich DM, O'Connor PJ, et al.: Improving diabetes care in practice: Findings from the TRANSLATE trial, *Diabetes Care* 31:2238-2243, 2008.

Sandison S: Negative pressure wound therapy promoted healing of diabetic foot ulcers more than advanced moist wound therapy, *Evidence-Based Nursing* 11:116, 2008.

Whittemore R: A multicomponent intervention improved diabetes care in primary care practices, *Evidence-Based Nursing* 12:89, 2009.

Answer Key

CHAPTER 1

Activity 1
1. c
2. b
3. d
4. a
5. g
6. e
7. f
8. h

Activity 2
1. a
2. a
3. b
4. b
5. a

Activity 3
1. b
2. b
3. a
4. b
5. a
6. a
7. b.

Activity 4
1. ideas, assumptions, principles, arguments, conclusions, beliefs, and actions
2. active; inner; the writer
3. three or four
4. Preliminary: comprehensive; analysis; synthesis
5. Preliminary
6. Comprehensive
7. Parts; whole

Activity 5
1. Yes
2. Yes
3. No
4. No
5. Yes; Self-Rated Abilities Scale for Health Practices (SRAHP)
6. Yes
7. Yes
   Summary: I would categorize this study as quantitative. It meets five of the seven criteria listed. It is a quasi-experimental, pretest-posttest study.

Activity 6
1. In order to base your practice on scientific evidence gained through research, you must first understand the research process. Then you need to know how to critique research in order to decide whether particular studies and their results have enough merit to change your practice.
2. Depth in nursing science will occur when a sufficient number of nurse researchers replicate and have consistent findings in a substantive area of inquiry. It is important that each study builds on prior studies, adding new variables or questions as the need arises.
3. If, for instance, your area of practice is psychiatric/mental health nursing with an emphasis on chemical dependency, you would like research findings demonstrating that nursing interventions related to "knowledge deficit regarding addiction" have an effect on the outcome of increased sobriety time for the addict or alcoholic.

Activity 8

1. a. Quantitative since it is a randomized controlled trial, Level II
   b. Qualitative since it is a phenomenological design, Level VI
2. Answers for this activity will vary depending on the research article chosen.

POSTTEST

1. Vary
2. a. Concepts: pain, disability
   b. Will vary for each student
   c. Will vary for each student, possibilities include the following: how was pain defined, and do you agree with that concept of pain? Does limitation in one item on a scale equal functional disability? How do the patients define functional disability?
3. a. Test a hypothesis; analyze themes or concepts
   b. Conducted; used

CHAPTER 2

Activity 1

1. f
2. b
3. d
4. a
5. c
6. e

Activity 2

1. Yes; Yes; Yes
2. Yes; Yes; No
3. Yes; Yes; Yes
4. Yes, No; Yes
5. Yes; No; Yes

Activity 3

1. a
2. a
3. b
4. a
5. b

Activity 4

1. a. Iron
   b. Iron status
2. a. Family-centered care (FCC)
   b. Health-related quality of life (HRQOL)

3. a. continuous albuterol (usual or high dose)
   b. peak flow
4. a. dental prophylaxes
   b. glycemic control
5. a. parenting
   b. blood pressure and heart rate

Activity 5

1. DH, Hr
2. NDH, Hr
3. NDH, Ho
4. DH, Hr
5. DH, Hr

Activity 6

1. Yes
2. Yes
3. Yes
4. Yes
5. Yes
6. Yes
7. Yes

Activity 7

1. P = children with long bone fractures in ED
   I = intranasal fentanyl
   C = intravenous morphine
   O = pain control
2. P = obese school-age children and their parents
   I = group intervention
   C = routine care
   O = weight loss
3. P = men after LRP
   I = none
   C = none
   O = experiences

POSTTEST

1. "The purpose of this study was to test the effectiveness of the Deaf Heart Health Intervention (DHHI) in increasing self-efficacy for health behaviors related to risk for cardiovascular disease (CVD) among culturally deaf adults" (Jones et al., 2007, p. 185).
2. Quantitative
3. a. Yes; b. Yes; c. Yes
4. P = culturally deaf adults; I = DHHI; C = usual care; O = self-efficacy
5. IV = DHHI
   DV = self-efficacy

6. Yes; "The study hypothesis was that culturally deaf adults who receive the DHHI would demonstrate greater self-efficacy for targeted health-related behaviors than deaf adults who did not receive the DHHI" (Jones et al., 2007, p. 188); directional

CHAPTER 3

Activity 1
1. Bandura's Social Cognitive Theory (Jones et al., 2007, p. 187)
2. Self-efficacy
3. Yes; "belief in one's ability to perform a certain task" (Jones et al., 2007, p. 187)
4. Yes; Self-Rated Abilities Scale for Health Practices (SRAHP), "Self-efficacy for the targeted health behaviors was measured with the SRAHP" (Jones et al., 2007, p. 188)

Activity 2
1. S
2. P
3. P
4. S
5. S
6. P
7. S

Activity 3
1. PR
2. NPR
3. PR
4. PR
5. NPR

Activity 4
1. 9
2. Approximately 177,000
3. CINAHL
4. CINAHL

Activity 5
1. a. Diets and behavioral interventions: effects on weight loss
   b. Lifestyle interventions: effects on maintenance of weight loss
   c. Lifestyle interventions for maintaining weight loss
2. a. Review: dietary intervention plus exercise is no better than dietary intervention alone for inducing long-term weight loss
   b. Review: dietary plus pharmacological intervention (orlistat or sibutramine) induces long-term weight loss in overweight or obese adults
   c. Review: dietary interventions, with or without exercise, promote weight loss more than advice alone
3. a. Exercise for type 2 diabetes mellitus
   b. Interventions to reduce weight gain in schizophrenia
   c. Multiple risk factor interventions for primary prevention of coronary heart disease
4. a. Intracellular lipid accumulation in liver and muscle and the insulin resistance syndrome
   b. Comprehensive clinical management of polycystic ovary syndrome
   c. The new "lower is better" lipid goals: are they achievable with today's drugs?
5. Although Evidence-Based Nursing retrieved preappraised single systematic reviews that provided applications for clinical practice in the commentary, Clinical Evidence also preappraised the evidence and provided a summary of multiple systematic reviews in the "Comment" section. Clinical Evidence provided the best available evidence for the clinical question. Note that, depending on the clinical question, other layers of the "5S" pyramid may provide the best available evidence for a particular clinical question.

Activity 6
1. Yes; includes review of literature on "Quality of Life and Breast Cancer" and "Cancer Treatment"
2. Not identified
3. Yes; examples of theoretical literature: (1) Meneses, K. (in review) and (2) Ferrell, Dow, and Grant (1995); examples of research literature: (1) Ashbury, Cameron, Mercer, Fitch, and Nielson (1998) and (2) Badger, Segrin, Meek, Lopez, and Bonham (2004)
4. Yes; Quality of Life (QOL)
5. Yes
6. Yes; "Only a small number of intervention studies in post-treatment survivorship have applied variations of psychoeducational and support interventions to reduce QOL-related issues" (Meneses et al., 2007, p. 1008)
7. No

8. Somewhat; does follow in a logical sequence but without consideration of the overall strengths and weaknesses of the reviewed studies to arrive at the logical conclusion.

9. Yes; clustered by topic, first "Quality of Life and Breast Cancer" and then "Cancer Survivorship Intervention Research," which is divided into "Intervention studies during active cancer treatment" and "Intervention studies during post-treatment survivorship"

10. Yes

11. Somewhat; does not explicitly state the research question(s) or hypotheses

POSTTEST

1. Cascade model (Kahana, Kahana, Namazi, Kercher, & Stange, 1997) and biocultural model (Bates, 1987)

2. (a) Pain; (b) functional disability; (c) race; (d) health conditions

3. No

4. No

5. Pain = single question, VDS, McGill Pain Questionnaire; Functional disability = SIP Short form; Race = single question; Health conditions = OARS Multidimensional Assessment

6. a. P, PR
   b. S, PR
   c. S, PR

7. Yes

8. Search strategy does not indicate the databases searched

9. Yes

10. Yes

11. Yes; "few published clinical studies on this topic have focused on samples of adults recruited from pain clinics, which limits generalizability. Very few researchers have examined relationships between pain and disability in Black and White older adults, and even fewer have controlled for socioeconomic and sociodemographic variables" (Horgas et al., 2008, p. 14).

12. No

13. No

14. Yes

15. Yes

16. Yes

CHAPTER 4

Activity 1

1. a. Quantitative research: The quantitative approach to research is based in the belief that we can best understand humans and their behavior by taking the human apart. We study specific characteristics one at a time. We measure each one as we go in the hopes that we can understand each characteristic in a clear and context-free manner. Once we clearly understand all of the pieces, we can put them together and understand the whole. Quantitative studies rely much more heavily on preselected instruments, collect lots of data, and answer questions through the analysis of numbers that represent those characteristics.

   b. Qualitative research: The qualitative approach to research is an accepted way to discover knowledge that uses naturalistic approaches to learn about human phenomena. This method of research is grounded in the social sciences and provides nurses with ways to better understand the lived experience and human processes that surround health and illness.

2. Homes, schools, hospitals, communities, outpatient settings, wherever people live every day

3. Explanatory or descriptive; words

Activity 2

a. Naturalistic setting: where people live every day; homes, schools, communities

b. Context: the place where something occurs and can include physical place, cultural beliefs, and life experience

c. Paradigm: from the Greek word meaning "pattern," it has come to describe how a person or a group of people think about the world

d. Purposive sample: nonprobability sampling where a researcher selects subjects considered typical of the population

e. Inclusion and exclusion criteria: limitations on eligibility or exclusion from a study population

f. Data saturation: point where enough data have been collected that the information being shared becomes repetitive, no new ideas are emerging

g. "Grand tour" question: a broad overview; may start with "tell me about…"

Activity 3
Review Appendix D (Landreneau & Ward-Smith, 2007)
Find and summarize the following elements:

	Landreneau & Ward-Smith, 2007
Purpose	The aim of this study was to explore what patients on hemodialysis perceive concerning choice among three types of renal replacement therapies: transplantation, hemodialysis, and peritoneal dialysis.
Design	An exploratory descriptive study
Sample and setting	A convenience sample of 20 patients was recruited from two urban dialysis units in the southern part of the United States. Interviews were conducted on the dialysis unit.
Methods	Phenomenological quantitative design, interviews were conducted following a script, interviews were taped and transcribed, data were analyzed using Colaizzi's framework.
Inclusion criteria	ESRD, over 18 years of age, hemodialysis therapy only for > 1 week, present at study site for more than one treatment, able to converse in and understand English.

Activity 4
Answers for this activity will vary depending on the research question chosen.

Activity 5: Web-Based Activity
(To complete this activity, you must read the essay titled "How Can We Argue for Evidence in Nursing?" at www.contemporarynurse.com/11.1/-1-1p5.htm.)

Consider what kinds of evidence you might need to adequately care for all the needs of a young woman with type 1 diabetes who has suffered the complications of blindness and kidney failure, and spends 3 days a week associating with very ill elderly individuals on dialysis. Although much of her care may be related to the hemodialysis and physiological responses of her body to this medical procedure, nurses are also concerned about the holistic needs of patients. What kinds of evidence do you think might be needed to enable a nurse to provide optimal or excellent care for this client? What kinds of evidence might you need to know about caregivers, the family household, adjusting to blindness, socialization needs, and other aspects of abilities to accomplish activities of daily living? What kinds of contributions might researchers using qualitative methods make to identify the kinds of interventions needed? The evidence that nurses need to provide optimal nursing care for the whole person may not be fully provided through quantitative studies. Qualitative research that explores the behavioral, emotional, and spiritual aspects of living with illness is needed so that we can truly identify what might be the best nursing approaches for meeting specific care needs. This is an area where nurses will make large contributions in the next few decades.

POSTTEST
1. a. Quantitative
   b. Quantitative
   c. Qualitative
   d. Quantitative
   e. Qualitative
   f. Quantitative
   g. Qualitative

h. Qualitative
i. Quantitative
j. Qualitative

2. Review of the literature: extensive, systematic, critical review of most important published scholarly literature on the topic

Study design: blueprint for a study

Sample: representative units from a population, description of process for selection

Setting for recruitment and data collection: description of where subjects were recruited and where data collection occurred

Data collection: description of how informed consent was obtained, what occurred between contact with the participant and the end of the interview, how were data collected, was a recording made, how long was the interview

Data analysis: how did the researcher take the raw data—words—and analyze them to find commonalities and differences; usually you will find an example

Findings: a presentation of the results, a description of the phenomenon, and the role or theme

CHAPTER 5

Activity 1

1. a. scientific; artistic
   b. natural settings
   c. day-to-day life
   d. lived experience
   e. less
   f. everyday living; human uniqueness
   g. research question
   h. fit
2. a. D
   b. A
   c. C
   d. F
   e. B
   f. I
   g. J
   h. G
   i. E
   j. H
3. a. Element 1: Identifying the phenomenon
   1. Phenomenology: study of day-to-day existence for a particular group of people

   2. Grounded theory method: interested in social processes from perspective of human interactions
   3. Ethnography: study of the complex cultural aspects related to a phenomenon
   4. Historical research: an approach for understanding a past event
   5. Case study: a focus on an individual, family, community, an organization, or some other complex phenomenon
   6. Community-based participatory research: a systematic study or assessment of a community to plan context-appropriate action
   b. Element 2: Structuring the study
   1. Phenomenology: Query the lived experience, research perspective is bracketed, sample has either lived or is living the experience being investigated.
   2. Grounded theory: Questions address basic social processes and tend to be action-oriented; researcher brings some knowledge of the literature but exhaustive review is not done before beginning the research. The researcher has concerns about contextual values and the data are the essence of the theory that emerges. The sample would be participants who have had experience with the circumstances, events, or incidents being studied.
   3. Ethnography: Questions are about lifeways or patterns of behavior within a social or cultural context. Researcher attempts to make sense of world from insider's point of view. The researcher becomes the interpreter of events and tries to make sense of and understand things from an emic point of view. Researchers do this by making their own beliefs explicit and set aside their own biases or assumptions in order to better understand a different world view. The sample often consists of key informants who have knowledge, status, and the communication skills needed to describe the phenomenon being studied.

4. Historical: Questions are implicit and embedded in the phenomenon studied; researcher understands information without imposing interpretation. It is important for the researcher to clearly and carefully identify the event(s) being studied. Data used for the study may be of a primary or secondary nature.

5. Case study: Questions about issues that serve as a foundation to uncover complexity and pursue understanding. The perspective of the researcher is reflected in the questions. Researchers may choose the most common cases or instead select the most unusual ones.

6. Community-based participatory research: Questions in this form of research are framed around the ideas of "look." Look has to do with identification of the stakeholders and understanding the problems from their perspective.

c. Element 3: Gathering the data
1. Phenomenology: written or oral data may be collected
2. Grounded theory: collect data through audiotaped and transcribed interviews and skilled observations
3. Ethnography: participant observation, immersion, informant interviews
4. Historical: use of primary and secondary data sources
5. Case study: use of interview, observations, document reviews, and other methods
6. Community-based participatory research: seeks to engage stakeholders in discovering the answers to the community problems

d. Element 4: Analyzing the data
1. Phenomenology: Move from the participant's description to the researcher's synthesis.
2. Grounded theory: Data collection and analysis occur simultaneously, use theoretical sampling, constant comparative method, and axial coding.
3. Ethnography: Data are collected and analyzed simultaneously, searching for symbolic categories.

4. Historical: Analyze for importance and then validity (authenticity) and reliability.
5. Case study: Reflecting and revising meanings.
6. Community-based participatory research: This stage of research is the "think" phase and is where what has been learned is interpreted or analyzed. The research has the role of linking the ideas provided by the stakeholders in an understandable way so that evidence for specific ways to address the problem can be provided to the community group.

e. Element 5: Describing the findings
1. Phenomenology: a narrative elaboration of the lived experience
2. Grounded theory: descriptive language to show theory connections to the data
3. Ethnography: large quantities of data; provide examples from the data and propositions about relationships of phenomena
4. Historical: well-synthesized chronicle
5. Case study: chronologically developed cases, a story that describes case dimensions or vignettes that emphasize various aspects of the case
6. Community-based participatory research: information obtained in earlier research stages sets the stage for community planning, implementation, and evaluation

4. Your answers may vary based on your personal interests. For example, a personal interest in the health behaviors of individuals and families in a culturally unique group might lead to the selection of an ethnographic method of investigation. This research method allows the investigator to explore multiple aspects of individual and family life, means of communication and behaviors, locations and substance of family households, the impact of the situated context where they reside, and other related factors. The health practices of a specific cultural group can be understood from emic and etic perspectives, ideas that may be similar or different. Data are collected through observation, interviews, identifying objects and their uses, and determining valu-

ing associated with symbols, behaviors, and objects.

Activity 2

1. The main theme of the literature review was costs for treatment with renal replacement vary significantly. Although there have been studies on the provider's perspective on renal replacement, the patient perspective has been missing. There have not been any studies to date addressing patient perspective of choice between three renal replacement therapies.

2. The literature review describes specific programs offering access to renal replacement, and differences in cost between therapies. The authors also describe a split between studies of dialysis therapy and transplant therapy. The authors make a case for understanding that there is a need for understanding why patients choose one renal replacement therapy over another.

3. The pilot study included all three groups, transplantation, renal dialysis, and peritoneal dialysis. The data gathered in the pilot study were too broad in scope. Thus, a follow-up larger qualitative study focused on only the hemodialysis patients since they had given the "richest descriptions" in the pilot study.

Activity 3

1. The research design used in this study was an exploratory descriptive study using a phenomenological approach to describe what patients on hemodialysis perceived of their choice of renal replacement therapies.

2. The authors used a purposive, convenience samples. A random sample of 20 patients was chosen from 175 patients on 2 hemodialysis units who had consented to be contacted again. The sample was selected based upon experience with hemodialysis and ability to share their knowledge.

3. The procedures used to collect data in this study were interviews following a open-ended guide that lasted from 30 to 45 minutes. Interviews were conducted on the dialysis unit. Interviews were taped and later transcribed verbatim within 2 weeks.

4. Phenomenological analysis using Coaizzi's framework was used to find beliefs, assumptions, and meaning. The researcher listened to the transcripts multiple times prior to tran-

scription. The researcher became immersed in the data to fully understand what was said. Meaning was extracted and data analysis showed that the words choice and knowledge were important themes. The researcher used a collaborative method with another nurse researcher to validate the formulated meanings and patients were asked to comment on the data themes and interpretations.

Activity 4

You may have some different ideas about the implications of this study for nursing practice, but here are a few things to consider:

- Knowledge is important to patients and patients may receive knowledge from many sources. Providing patients with outdated or inaccurate information could influence their treatment choice and may lead to more risks or costs to the patient as well as reduced benefits from treatment. Choice is important to patients. In this study the authors found that even when patients had limited participation in the decision for a specific renal replacement therapy, they perceived that they had a choice. Informed choice based on accurate information provides the best chance for patients to make a decision based on all options, not just the treatment offered initially.

- Rising rates of hypertension, diabetes, and obesity will increase the number of people with ESRD. How do you think the increasing costs of ESRD will be dealt with in the future? Can you see areas where improvement in nursing care could lead to better patient outcomes and decreased costs for treatment?

Activity 5

a. D
b. C
c. B
d. A
e. A
f. B
g. E
h. C
i. D
j. D
k. A
l. C
m. E
n. C

o. D

p. C

q. B

r. A

s. E

t. A (could also be true of B or C)

u. A (could also be true of B, C, or D)

v. C

w. D (could also be true of A or C)

x   C (could also be true of A)

y. B

z. B

Activity 6

Answers for this activity will vary depending on the research question chosen.

Activity 7: Web-Based Activity

Qualitative research provides many unique ways to add to nursing's body of knowledge as it supplies evidence related to the complex behavioral relationships between humans and humans with their environment. This activity is intended to expose you to the broad kinds of investigation being done using qualitative research.

Answers for this activity will vary depending on the research question chosen.

POSTTEST

1. T

2. T

3. F

4. T

5. F

6. a

7. d

8. b

9. a

10. d

11. c

12. e

13. a, b, d, or f

14. c

CHAPTER 6

Activity 1

The primary theme of this first discussion of the findings describes examples of knowledge about what renal replacement therapy does for their body, what the conditions for each replacement therapy were, and when the information was given to patients and who presented that information. The quotations included illustrate patient understanding and provide insight into how and where patients learned about renal replacement.

Activity 2

1. This study found that this group of renal replacement patients described having a "choice" of treatment even when their participation in deciding on a treatment was often minimal. Often patient knowledge of renal replacement was inaccurate and may have led to treatment choices that were not medically optimal.

2. The authors state that this study is a first step in understanding perception of choice in renal replacement therapy. This study is helping to create a new body of knowledge, but the authors caution that additional research will be required. This study should not be generalized to other patient populations.

3. Patient knowledge came from many sources, from different medical doctors, from dialysis nurses, and even from people on the street. Information was given to patients at a variety of times during treatment. Participants in this study provided statements about their knowledge of renal replacement therapies that were medically inaccurate.

4. There are many possibilities for future research. This list is not exhaustive; there are many other potential studies:

    A study on the order of replacement therapies presented to patients and the impact of this order on treatment choice.

    A study on patient perceptions of choice and knowledge of renal replacement therapy for hemodialysis, peritoneal dialysis, and renal transplant patients.

    A study of staff perceptions of risk for the different renal replacement therapies among transplant surgeons, nephrologists, dialysis nurses, etc.

    A survey of renal replacement patients to assess the amount of medically inaccurate beliefs about the renal replacement therapies that they are not receiving.

Activity 3

1. a. G

    b. B

    c. D
    d. A
    e. F
    f. D
    g. E
    h. G
    i. B

2. a. *Credibility* refers to qualitative research steps taken to ensure the accuracy, validity, and soundness of the data. Credibility can be confirmed when the research participants recognize the reported findings as their personal experience.

    b. *Auditability* is a research process that allows the work of a qualitative researcher or a person critiquing a research report to follow the thinking and/or conclusions of a researcher. The question of concern is whether the researcher(s) presented enough information for the reader to clearly understand the ways data were interpreted. When a data trail is auditable, it leads to the possibility of confirmability or an ability to clearly understand the ways the data were obtained, analyzed, and interpreted.

    c. *Fittingness* is the term used to answer these three questions: Are the findings applicable outside the study? Are the results or feelings meaningful to people not involved in the research? Are the findings meaningful to others who are in similar situations? Another idea closely related to fittingness is *transferability;* can the findings be translated into similar experiences in meaningful ways?

    d. *Saturation* refers to the point where data are being replicated in ways where no new ideas are coming forth about a specific concept or cultural phenomenon.

    e. *Trustworthiness* implies that validity and reliability have been established and when a research report accurately represents or portrays the participants' experience.

Activity 4: Web-Based Activity

Your instructor may want to direct you to view some specific Internet links to learn additional specific aspects of qualitative research.

POSTTEST
1. F
2. F
3. T
4. T
5. T
6. F
7. Auditability
8. Generalizability
9. Credibility
10. Creditability, auditability, fittingness

CHAPTER 7

Activity 1
1. h
2. j
3. e
4. g
5. d
6. f
7. b
8. a
9. c

Activity 2
1. Testing. Taking the test repeatedly may be the factor leading to an increase in confidence and accuracy, rather than the experimental program. The use of different outcome instruments and measures may be necessary.
2. Instrumentation. The use of standardized calibrated equipment and training for the volunteers would increase the internal validity of the findings.
3. History. The increase in taxes could account for a decrease in the rate of cigarette smoking. Use of a control group and randomization would improve interpretation of the findings.
4. Selection bias. The difference between groups is difficult to assess because the participants self-selected themselves into the treatment or control group.
5. Mortality. The program is not successful for single homeless women with preschool children. It is important to look at the makeup of the final study sample when the results are interpreted.
6. Maturation. The mothers' confidence could be increased by any number of factors, including the act of caring for their infant during the

month. The time of measurement could be immediately before discharge. Use of a control group would strengthen the findings.

Activity 3

a. The setting consisted of small group meetings with 5 to 10 people at community locations in Phoenix and Tucson.

b. The subjects were 105 deaf adults recruited in Phoenix and Tucson, Arizona.

c. The investigators outlined two criteria for participant selection: 18 years or older and self-identification as a member of deaf culture.

d. People under 18 years of age and people with a previous diagnosis of CVD were excluded from the study.

e. No, the sample could not be randomly assigned to control and intervention groups because of the threat of "cross-talk." The groups differed in ethnic composition.

f. Instruments were the Self-Rated Abilities Scale for Health Practices (SRAHP). Demographic data and scores for the subsections of the SRAHP were collected. The intervention group in Tucson received the Deaf Heart Health Intervention (DHHI), and the control group in Phoenix had an alternate treatment that consisted of the same number of hours of social activities. All sessions were held in small groups of 5 to 10 people in community settings for both groups. The PI visited the DHHI sessions to ensure fidelity.

g. The group in Phoenix served as the control group because more of the research team lived in Tucson.

Activity 4

1. Yes, the design is appropriate. The investigators were interested in evaluating the effectiveness of a psychoeducational program on quality of life for breast cancer survivors and used a randomized controlled trial to do this.

2. Yes, the methods used for control are consistent with the research design. Control is managed by ruling out extraneous or mediating variables that would compete with the independent variables as an explanation for a study's outcome. Meneses et al. maintain control of extraneous variables by using a wait control group, research team training, a protocol manual, tape recording of all education sessions with random viewing of 20% of sessions, monthly team meetings, homogeneous sample, consistent data collection procedures, and manipulation of the independent variable and randomization of the sample into groups by a biostatistician.

3. Time: the study took 6 months to collect the data. Subject availability: this study used outpatient breast cancer survivors. Equipment required included questionnaires, telephones, written materials, tape recordings, etc.

4. Yes, the parts of the study fit together and there is a logical flow to the design. The clinical concern and intervention is supported by the literature, which links to the research objective and leads to the chosen design.

5. Threats to internal validity include history, maturation, instrumentation, mortality, and selection bias. The authors explained effectively how they controlled for maturation.

   History—The authors note no unanticipated events during the course of the study. This is difficult to evaluate because we are not given the dates when the study took place.

   Maturation—The authors note that perceptions about illness and state of physical well-being may have affected participant's quality of life over the course of the study. The wait-control group helped to control for this by providing a natural history of the course of survivorship without psychoeducational intervention.

   Instrumentation—There is no reason to think that the instruments changed during the course of the study.

   Mortality—The investigators report that retention in this study was 98%, with 256 of 261 women completing the study. One participant in the control group died of a noncancer cause during the study.

   Selection bias—Meneses et al. established criteria for selection of subjects and had an experimental and a control group.

6. Threats to external validity include selection, reactive effects, and measurement effects.

   Selection—Meneses et al. note that their sample was comprised predominantly of Caucasian English-speaking females with college degrees.

   Reactive effects—It is possible that there could have been some positive outcomes simply from being included in the study and receiving monthly telephone calls.

Measurement effects—The instruments that were given at more than one point in the study were the Breast Cancer Treatment and Sociodemographic Data Tool and the Quality of Life–Breast Cancer Survivor scale (used at baseline, 3 months, and 6 months).

Activity 5: Web-Based Activity
It is possible to ascertain from the titles whether a study was most likely qualitative or quantitative. Results will depend on the year selected. However, this is an excellent site to learn about the most current funded research studies that are taking place. If you find a topic that is of interest to you, you may want to look for an article by the author, or if it is not yet published, you could contact the author because his or her university affiliation is listed.

Activity 6: Evidence-Based Practice Activity
1. Meta-analysis of RCTs; C
2. A well-designed RCT; C
3. Quasi-experimental study; C
4. Single nonexperimental study; C
5. Systematic review of qualitative studies; B, C
6. Single descriptive or qualitative study; A
7. Opinion of authorities, report of expert committee; A, E

POSTTEST
1. a. Purpose: To examine the effectiveness of a psychoeducational program on quality of life in breast cancer survivors
    b. Academic center and regional cancer center in the southwest United States
    c. Breast cancer survivors, >21 years old, stage 0–11 breast cancer without metastasis or local recurrence, within 1 year of diagnosis, who had surgery, radiation, and/or chemo at least 1 month before, spoke English, and were able to participate
    d. Randomly assigned to treatment or wait control
    e. The BCEI
    f. Random assignment to groups, study design, interventionist training, intervention delivery, procedure manual, didactic training in BCEI, tape recording of sessions, monthly team meetings, participant evaluation of the BCEI

2. a. Control
    b. Accuracy
    c. External validity
    d. Maturation
    e. Feasibility
    f. Internal validity
    g. Selection bias

CHAPTER 8

Activity 1
1. Experimental
2. Solomon four-group design
3. Time series design
4. After-only experiment
5. After-only nonequivalent control group design
6. True experimental
7. Nonequivalent control group design

Activity 2
1. Quasi-experimental, pretest-posttest design.
2. Subjects cannot be assigned to groups randomly, thus it is a quasi-experimental design. The lack of randomization may lead to threats to internal validity.
3. a. Antecedent variables include ethnicity, age, education, gender, living situation, and marital status. The authors note that the difference in ethnicity between the two sites was significant and could be a threat to internal validity.
    b. Intervening variables include increased exercise, change in diet, relaxation, or other health-related behavior change during the experiment that was not related to the DHHI.
4. The evidence provided by the findings of the study shows the promise of the DHHI to help reduce health disparities in deaf Americans. Further research will be required to determine the ability of the DHHI to reduce CVD risk. Further study will be required to examine the relationships among ethnicity, SES, health-related self-efficacy, and health behaviors in the deaf community.

Activity 3

1.

	Pretest	Teaching	Posttest
Group A	X	X	X
Group B		X	X
Group C	X		X
Group D			X

Note: The groups may be arranged in any order, but the four-group pattern must be followed.

2. The nurses would be randomly assigned to each of the groups using a table of random numbers or computer random assignment.
3. The pain knowledge and attitudes questionnaire would be used as a pretest.
4. The teaching program is the experimental treatment.
5. The pain knowledge and attitudes questionnaire is also the posttest or outcome measure.
6. The Solomon four-group design is ideal for experimental studies in which the pretest might affect the outcome. In this case, the questionnaire might change nurses' knowledge and attitudes about pain management. The researcher will be able to compare results for nurses receiving the teaching and not receiving the teaching with and without the pretest.
7. This type of design is particularly effective in ruling out threats to internal validity that the before-and-after groups may experience. It is effective for highly sensitive issues, which might be affected by simply completing a questionnaire as a baseline pretest.
8. A disadvantage of the Solomon four-group design is that a large number of subjects must be available for assignment into the four groups.

Activity 4

1. a. Other potential designs are true experimental, Soloman four, or after only. These tests would require conditions other than the conditions the authors were working with in the study. The authors chose a quasi-experimental, pretest-posttest design because of the potential for "cross-talk" among deaf individuals living in the same city. The authors chose not to randomize participants to experimental and control groups to prevent contact between control and intervention groups in this tight-knit community. Additionally, the researchers lived nearer to one site than the other and this helped with supervision of the intervention group.
   b. The presence of a pretest allows the investigator to compare the two groups on important antecedent variables before the intervention (treatment variable) is implemented.
   c. The small sample size, lack of randomization, and differences between the control and intervention groups led to questions about the effect of the DHHI. Additionally, the effect of demographic characteristics on the results of the SRAHP following the DHHI cannot be determined.
2. a. Randomized controlled trial
   b. All subjects in both control and intervention groups received the same "attention" from the research team (including phone calls and face-to-face interaction). The control group did receive the same psychoeducational support and educational sessions *after* measuring the differences between groups for 6 months. This method allows the patients to all receive educational support, but allows the researchers control and the ability to measure the effect of the intervention (measurement of causation) apart from simply paying attention to the participants.

c. Overall quality of life, physical, psychological, social, and spiritual well-being
d. Breast Cancer Education Intervention (BCEI)

Activity 5
1. Quasi-experimental designs may be more practical, more feasible, and more adaptable to real-world practice. In many studies important to nursing, it is not possible to randomize subjects into groups for practical or ethical reasons.
2. The researcher must carefully examine other factors that could account for differences between groups.
3. The clinician must carefully critique the research study and also look for other factors, which might explain the results of the study. The results of any study with any design must be evaluated to determine if other factors influence the findings. The results should also be compared with the findings of other similar studies.

Activity 6: Web-Based Activity
1. This number will vary depending on when the search is conducted.
2. The types of articles will vary depending on when the search is conducted, but often you will find editorials, review articles, and research studies.
3. This number will vary depending on when the search is conducted.
4. This number will vary depending on when the search is conducted.

Activity 7: Evidence-Based Practice Activity
1. Level 3
2. Level 2

POSTTEST
1. a. E
   b. Q
   c. E
   d. E
   e. Q
2. a. 3
   b. 1
   c. 2
   d. 6
   e. 4
   f. 5

CHAPTER 9

Activity 1

L	**O**	**N**	**G**	**I**	**T**	**U**	**D**	**I**	**N**	**A**	**L**	**D**	**M**	**E**
C	I	S	P	U	E	Q	W	H	X	O	I	**Y**	H	**X**
C	**R**	F	L	G	Y	Q	E	R	C	X	**E**	**C**	G	**P**
U	W	**O**	L	Z	S	B	Q	F	H	**V**	**O**	H	H	**O**
N	T	L	**S**	C	I	S	Z	A	**R**	**R**	O	I	U	**S**
L	G	T	R	**S**	D	L	D	**U**	**R**	Z	L	D	O	**T**
U	E	I	O	I	**S**	Q	**S**	**E**	D	L	V	W	O	**F**
I	U	W	S	J	J	**E**	**L**	O	S	Y	U	H	I	**A**
G	T	D	K	X	O	**A**	**C**	I	E	M	D	I	I	**C**
Q	W	R	E	E	**T**	O	K	**T**	T	E	S	T	A	**T**
A	S	A	M	**I**	K	E	N	B	**I**	B	H	U	L	**O**
D	U	O	**O**	K	L	H	N	P	H	**O**	B	Z	V	F
M	C	**N**	G	U	L	U	E	O	L	Y	**N**	R	K	C
K	**A**	M	F	G	U	P	Q	S	B	Z	L	**A**	H	T
L	W	J	F	V	N	E	W	J	S	W	L	E	**L**	V

1. Survey
2. Longitudinal
3. Correlational
4. Ex post facto
5. Cross-sectional
6. Correlational
7. Longitudinal
8. Survey
9. Cross-sectional
10. Cross-sectional

Activity 2

	Advantages	Disadvantages
Correlation studies	A3	D1, D3, D4, D7
Cross-sectional	A1, A8	D2, D5
Ex post facto	A4	D1, D2, D3, D4, D5, D7
Longitudinal	A2, A6	D2, D8, D9
Prospective	A2, A7	D3, D4, D7, D8
Retrospective	A4	D1, D2, D3, D4, D5, D7
Survey	A1	D5, D7

Activity 3
1 Exploratory survey
2. Longitudinal, or prospective
3. Cross-sectional
4. Retrospective or ex post facto
5. Correlational
6. Methodological
7. Meta-analysis

Activity 4
1. Meta-analysis
2. Yes: studies had to have at least two treatment groups, subject placement in groups had to be random; studies with historical controls were excluded.
3. Under "Search Methods," dates were 1983–July 2007; "nurse," "health visitor," "nursing," "smoking cessation"
4. Assessment of selection bias, performance bias, attrition bias, and detection bias was made using the Cochrane Handbook. A three-point scale was used to grade the studies.

Activity 5
Ex post facto design

Activity 6: Web-Based Activity
1. Answers for this activity will vary depending on when the search is conducted.
2. Answers for this activity will vary depending on when the search is conducted.

Activity 7: Evidence-Based Practice Activity
1. d
2. b
3. a, b

POSTTEST
1. Variables
2. Survey
3. Descriptive, exploratory, comparative
4. Relationship-difference
5. Correlational
6. Interrelational
7. Retrospective
8. a. Cross-sectional
   b. Longitudinal/prospective
   c. Retrospective/ex post facto
9. Cross sectional; longitudinal
10. Prospective
11. Retrospective
12. Methodological

CHAPTER 10

Activity 1
1. Sample: Set of units that are selected to represent an entire population.
   Population: Well-defined set that has certain specified properties, may be defined broadly or narrowly.
   Differences: The population is the entire set of units with specified characteristics. The entire population is not often feasible to include in a study. The sample is a subset of the population that is selected to represent the entire population.
2. Target Population: The entire population that meets the sampling criteria.
   Accessible Population: A population that meets the target population criteria and that is available to the researcher.
   Differences: The target population is the whole, whereas the accessible population is the slice that is available to the researcher.
3. Inclusion criteria: Population descriptors used to select a sample.
   Exclusion criteria: Characteristics that restrict the population to make it more homogeneous.
   Differences: These terms describe the same concept. Inclusion, exclusion, eligibility, and delimitations are all terms used to describe subject attributes that researchers consider when determining if the individual is part of a population.

Activity 2
1. Probability sampling uses random selection and is more rigorous. Nonprobability sampling uses nonrandom methods and there is no way to ensure that each element has a chance for inclusion in the sample.
2. a. N
   b. N
   c. P
   d. N
   e. P
   f. P

Activity 3
1. b
2. d
3. a
4. c

5. d
6. e
7. d

Activity 4

1. a. Yes, the sample is adequately described. The inclusion criteria were noted as patients who were at least 21 years old, histologically confirmed breast cancer stage 0–II with no evidence of local recurrence or metastatic disease, within 1 year of diagnosis, had surgery, radiation, or chemotherapy at least 1 month prior, were able to communicate in English, and were able to participate.
    b. No, all women with breast cancer were not included in the study. The population demographics of the sample may not reflect the demographics of the entire population with breast cancer. Patients with local recurrence or metastatic disease were not included in the sample.
    c. Simple random
    d. Probability
    e. 261 women participated, 5 women did not complete the study. 256 women completed the study. The retention rate was 98%.
2. Sample selection is not subject to biases of researcher, sample representativeness is maximized, probability of choosing a nonrepresentative sample is decreased.
3. Method is time consuming. It may be very difficult to have a listing of every element in the population.
4. Random selection of subjects is more rigorous than nonprobability sampling and the sample is more likely to represent the population of interest. Risk of bias is reduced.

Activity 5

1. True
2. True
3. False
4. False
5. True
6. True
7. False

Activity 6

1. Yes, the characteristics of the sample were well described.

2. Yes, the parameters of the population for this study would be community-dwelling seniors present at senior centers and churches in a city in the Midwest in 2000.
3. The sample may not be representative of community dwelling older Black and White adults. The choice of a convenience sample makes bias more likely.
4. The criteria were ≥60 years old, willing to participate, able to provide informed consent.
5. Based on the material provided in the article, you could answer yes. The delimitation or exclusion criteria specified participants who could not explain the study or provide informed consent, or if they were not able to complete the survey.
6. Yes, it may be possible to replicate the study sample if there were similar populations available in the proposed study geographic areas.
7. The sample was obtained from the populations of five senior centers and two churches in a large, diverse, Midwest city. Yes, the method was appropriate for a convenience sample for a descriptive/comparative survey design.
8. A convenience sample introduces more bias than any other sampling method, samples may not be representative of the population.
9. The sample size appears appropriate for this study. The authors state "several guidelines in the literature indicate that the sample size of the current analysis ($N = 115$) was sufficient for the relatively simple measurement and structural regression models" (p. 6).
10. Yes, approval was obtained from the institutional review board of the two institutions where data were collected and analyzed. In accordance with the consent process, if participants had difficulty completing the survey due to reasons other than physical disability (for instance, for writing difficulties), they were thanked for their time and the survey was discontinued. Participants were compensated $10.00 on completion of the survey.
11. Yes, they defined the limitations of this study. They mentioned that race was measured by racial category but not by ethnicity, the sample was of modest size, a convenience sample was used, sampling was limited to a few centers in a single city, participants were limited to those able to participate in community activities, the sample was nonrandom and may not have

represented the older adult population. Also, participants were not asked about pain medications that may have affected their responses to study questions.

Activity 7: Web-Based Activity
1. Answer will depend on state chosen and census year.
2. Answer will depend on state chosen and census year
3. **"White.** A person having origins in any of the original peoples of Europe, the Middle East, or North Africa. It includes people who indicate their race as 'White' or report entries such as Irish, German, Italian, Lebanese, Near Easterner, Arab, or Polish."
   "Black or African American. A person having origins in any of the Black racial groups of Africa. It includes people who indicate their race as 'Black, African Am., or Negro,' or provide written entries such as African American, Afro American, Kenyan, Nigerian, or Haitian."
4. The sample was 52% Black, 48% white, was also 77% female and 23% male. Comparisons between Table 1 in the study and census data will depend on the state chosen and the year of the census data.

Activity 8: Evidence-Based Practice Activity
The sample and sampling strategy is one variable that will influence the strength of the evidence provided by the study. The evidence from a meta-analysis of all *randomized* controlled trials is more influential in making practice change decisions than from a single descriptive or qualitative study with a convenience sample.

POSTTEST
1. Power analysis
2. Probability; nonprobability
3. Convenience
4. Simple random
5. Table of random numbers
6. Stratified random
7. Inclusion, exclusion criteria
8. Convenience, quota, purposive
9. Multistage or cluster
10. Data saturation

CHAPTER 11

Activity 1
1. Nursing research committee
2. Institutional review board
3. Justice
4. Expedited review
5. Unethical research study
6. HIPAA

Activity 2
1. Beneficence
2. Justice
3. Respect for person

Activity 3
Elements of Informed Consent
1. √ Title of protocol
2. √ Invitation to participate
3. 0 Basis for subject selection
4. √ Overall purpose of the study
5. √ Explanation of benefits
6. √ Description of risks and discomforts
7. √ Potential benefits
8. 0 Alternatives to participation
9. √ Financial obligations
10. √ Assurance of confidentiality
11. 0 In case of injury compensation
12. 0 HIPAA disclosure
13. √ Subject withdrawal
14. √ Offer to answer questions
15. √ Concluding consent statement
16. √ Identification of investigators

Activity 4
1. The elderly
2. Children
3. Pregnant women
4. The unborn
Other correct responses include those who are emotionally or physically disabled, prisoners, the deceased, students, and people with AIDS.

Activity 5
1. a, c, d, f, g
2. a, b, c, d, f, g (Also, presume "e" was not adhered to because the study began in 1932 before IRBs and formal consent were required.)

Activity 6
1. Appendix A, Meneses et al., in the "Procedure" section under "Methods," write,

"Following study approval by the respective institutional review board of the university where the researchers were affiliated at the time of the study and the participating cancer centers, potential subjects were identified by the cancer center or private oncology office nursing staff using an eligibility checklist …A staff member briefly explained the study and determined interest…Subjects expressing interest signed a consent form…upon receipt of the consent form, the BCEI project director followed up with potential subjects, explained the study objectives and time commitment, and answered any questions." The authors demonstrate that they obtained informed consent and approval by the IRB.

2. Appendix B, Horgas et al., document in the "Method" and "Procedure" sections of the article that institutional review board approval was obtained from the two appropriate institutions where data were collected and analyzed for the study. Additional protections for the elderly subjects were that patients were excluded if they could not explain the study after a description was given by a staff member or if they were unable to complete the survey.

3. Appendix C, Jones et al., report in the "Method" section under the heading "Sample" that "the study was approved by the University of Arizona Institutional Review Board for Protection of Human Subjects prior to subject recruitment." An additional protection for the subjects was that "the consent form was translated into ASL, presented to potential participants on video tape, and any questions were answered in sign language as part of the consenting procedure."

4. Appendix D, Landreneau et al., note in the "Data Collection" section of the article that "with the approval of the university internal review board for the protection of human subjects, approval from the dialysis units' internal review board, and permission of both dialysis units, the researcher approached 190 patients on hemodialysis from the 2 dialysis units and invited them to participate."

Activity 7: Web-Based Activity

1. National Cancer Institute
2. Yes, because it is a government Web site supported by the U.S. National Institutes of Health

Activity 8: Evidence-Based Practice Activity

You could check the *Federal Register* or other government documents or Web sites to determine if misconduct had occurred, or check the journal for a correction or follow-up research report.

POSTTEST

1. Yes, because extra precautions should be taken to protect the rights of vulnerable populations but this would not preclude undertaking research.
2. Before
3. Informed consent documents, IRB approval from the appropriate agency
4. Yes
5. Informed consent
6. Risks to subjects may be greater than benefits, a patient's basic human rights could be violated, and results of a study would be questionable.

CHAPTER 12

Activity 1
Study 1 (Meneses et al.)
1. d
2. Two instruments were used, the Breast Cancer Treatment and Sociodemographic Data Tool and the Quality of Life–Breast Cancer Survivors (QOL). The former tool captures treatment data and sociodemographic data, and allowed the researchers to analyze potential confounding variables in the data analysis. The QOL scale measures four domains of quality of life and was used to measure the effect of the intervention over time. Questionnaires allow self-report data to be collected; measuring quality of life could not be accomplished through physiological instruments. Questionnaires are particularly useful for collecting data on experiences, feelings, behaviors, or attitudes.

Study 2 (Jones et al.)
1. d
2. Self-efficacy is a belief in one's ability to perform a task. Beliefs cannot be observed or measured through physiological data. Beliefs can be measured through a questionnaire such as the Self-Rated Abilities Scale for

Health Practices, which measures self-efficacy in nutrition, psychological well-being/stress management, physical activity/exercise, and health practices.

3. It is believed to have been a successful data-collection method. The instruments were modified for administration in signed ASL or written form. The original written SRAHP and the signed version were tested to ensure that scores correlated and that internal consistency was maintained.

Study 3 (Horgas et al.)

1. d
2. The researchers wanted to understand the relationship between race, pain and disability. Several questionnaires were used to measure variables, including the following: verbal descriptor scale for pain, functional disability by the SIP Short Form, demographic data, and health conditions by the Older Americans Resources and Services Multidimensional Assessment. The questionnaires provided data that could be analyzed using structural equation modeling to look at the relationships between the study's main variables—pain, disability, and race. Other measures could not provide the self-report data required for this study.

Study 4 (Landreneau et al.)

1. c, d
2. The potential issues with self-reported data are social desirability and respondent burden. When participants want to answer questions in a socially desirable way, there is no way for researchers to know if they are telling the truth; therefore the accuracy of these measures is always open to question. Respondent burden can occur when surveys are too long or questions are too difficult for participants to answer given their age, health, or mental status. Being cognizant of the participant's ability to answer questions, keeping survey or interview time within reason, and choosing an instrument carefully can help reduce respondent fatigue.

Activity 2

1. Consumers
2. Physiological
3. Reactivity
4. Interviews
5. Records
6. Questionnaire
7. Objectivity, consistency
8. Concealment
9. Interrater reliability
10. Operationalization
11. Likert scale
12. Content analysis
13. Fun

D	E	L	I	V	E	R	S	T	A	T	I	S	T	C	S	Y	E	S	P	A	S
S	S	A	C	A	B	I	N	E	T	F	O	R	K	A	Z	O	S	P	E	I	O
I	A	W	O	P	E	R	A	T	I	O	N	A	L	I	Z	A	T	I	O	N	B
G	T	S	N	O	R	N	E	V	E	R	B	Y	D	N	E	A	U	X	B	T	J
N	S	Y	S	T	E	M	A	T	I	C	A	J	H	T	B	S	D	V	S	E	E
I	F	L	I	K	E	R	T	S	C	A	L	E	E	R	R	O	Y	A	E	R	C
F	A	K	S	C	A	L	E	S	N	O	V	N	O	C	A	A	U	L	R	R	T
H	C	U	T	A	C	R	A	T	I	M	A	P	V	E	T	P	U	I	V	A	I
Y	T	B	E	B	H	I	R	T	E	M	A	H	V	W	K	I	C	D	A	T	V
P	C	O	N	T	E	N	T	A	N	A	L	Y	S	I	S	P	V	O	T	E	I
R	O	Y	C	B	K	D	S	I	S	R	T	S	A	D	V	A	N	E	I	R	T
E	R	E	Y	O	D	U	G	K	A	T	P	I	B	I	O	I	O	G	O	R	Y
A	V	S	I	B	R	Q	U	E	S	T	I	O	N	N	A	I	R	E	N	E	C
C	I	A	R	E	S	E	A	R	C	H	L	L	R	E	A	C	E	S	O	L	O
T	O	B	M	E	X	C	E	L	A	E	O	O	D	A	T	A	C	O	V	I	N
I	U	E	A	E	V	A	L	I	D	S	T	G	N	O	S	T	O	O	E	A	S
V	N	Y	E	S	S	I	N	T	E	R	V	I	E	W	S	A	R	F	R	B	U
I	H	A	P	P	I	E	N	E	S	S	P	C	A	T	A	G	D	U	N	I	M
T	X	C	I	T	E	D	E	L	P	H	I	A	T	O	T	P	S	N	V	L	E
Y	C	E	A	T	U	B	B	S	A	N	D	L	D	O	N	N	M	A	R	I	R
Y	A	B	L	E	A	C	O	N	C	E	A	L	M	E	N	T	O	O	T	T	S
A	I	K	E	V	A	L	I	K	E	I	I	A	B	C	O	N	S	U	M	Y	S

Activity 3

1. Children; interactions between people where the investigator is not part of the interaction; psychiatric patients; classrooms
2. The consent is usually of the type where permission to observe for a specified purpose is requested. The specific behaviors that are to be observed are not named. The use of the data and degree of anonymity are explained. In some situations, the subjects will be asked to review the data after the observation and before inclusion in the data pool.
3. Reactivity is the major concern, when the investigator has reason to believe that his or her presence will change the nature of the subjects' behavior.

Activity 4

Physiological measures would be of minimal use since the data being sought would not involve actual measures of the residents' physiological status. Not particularly interested in current blood pressure, temperature, urinary output, etc.

Could consider using observation; for example, sitting in an emergency department and observing the types of health care concerns that enter. Would need to think about whether this would be observation with concealment. Would need to wrestle with the notion of what is private information and what is public domain information.

Could use questionnaires and collect data from all types of health care providers. Could provide a lot of data in a short time. Wonder how busy they would be and what would be the probability of their filling out the questionnaire?

Could use an interview. Is costly in terms of researcher time, but could provide more detailed information because subjects could be asked to expand on specific items. But who should be interviewed? How does one get into their offices/homes, etc.?

Need to get some information from the people who actually live here. How could you reach a cross section of the residents of your rural community? Could they be called? What about those people without a telephone?

Better check out the census data to get a clearer picture of what is being dealt with. Probably have some morbidity and mortality data collected by the state health department. Would probably use existing records to get a first sense of what the parameters of "health" are in this community. Then talk to some people about who knew the most about this area and arrange some interviews with these individuals. These would be guided interviews with open-ended items to encourage the sharing of as much information as possible. Would also seek a way to collect data from a variety of health care users; for example, surveys in the waiting room of various agencies, maybe the crowd at a mall, at a county fair.

One data collection instrument would not be sufficient to collect the information needed about the areas addressed.

Activity 5
1. d
2. a
3. d
4. a, b, c
5. d

Activity 6: Web-Based Activity
Answers will vary depending on when the search is conducted and what database is used.

Activity 7: Evidence-Based Practice Activity
Answers will vary depending on the topic chosen, when the search is conducted, and what database is used.

POSTTEST
1. d
2. d
3. c
4. b
5. b
6. d
7. c
8. d
9. b
10. b
11. b
12. d
13. a
14. d
15. a

CHAPTER 13

Activity 1
1. S; avoided by proper calibration of the scale.
2. S; decrease error by providing instructions, ensuring confidentiality, or other means to allow students to freely express themselves.
3. R; lessen by training research assistants and using strict protocols or rule books to guide analysis.
4. R; decrease their anxiety by addressing their concerns, providing comfort measures, or other efforts that might decrease their anxiety. Anxiety may alter the test responses.

Activity 2
1. Construct validity
2. Face validity
3. Concurrent validity
4. Context experts
5. Construct validity or convergent validity
6. Convergent validity; contrasted groups; divergent validity; factor analysis; hypothesis testing
7. Contrasted groups

Activity 3
1. Stability; homogeneity; equivalence
2. Test-retest methods could be accomplished by giving the same test again at a later date and seeing if the two scores are highly correlated. Parallel or alternate forms, such as alternate versions of the same test, could also be used to establish stability.
3. Alternate forms would be better if the test-taker is likely to remember and be influenced by the items or the answers from the first test.
4. a. 2
   b. 4
   c. 1
   d. 3
5. a. Yes, these instruments had face validity. The researchers were addressing functional disability in older adults. The information given about the SIP appears to measure disability.
   b. Was developed to measure physical and social disability. Was reported to be valid

and reliable, but was burdensome to complete.

c. The information provided for the instruments would increase confidence in the results of the study. Based on the descriptions, the instruments chosen were appropriate. If a greater understanding of the instruments is needed, the original articles referenced in this study would be a good place to start. Additional studies of the measures used could also provide information on recent changes or adaptations of the measures.

Activity 4
1. Healthy days are summarized per month as the number of days with good mental and physical health. Plus a symptom module that measures pain, depression, anxiety, sleeplessness, vitality, and activity limitation.
2. Medical Outcomes Study Short Form (SF-36)

Activity 5
1. Two instruments, the Breast Cancer Treatment and Sociodemographic Data Tool and the Quality of Life–Breast Cancer Survivors
2. a. No information on validity was given
   b. Test-retest reliability, Cronbach's alpha
   c. Yes, the test-retest allowed sufficient time between tests and the score was 0.89; Cronbach's alpha was >0.70 (0.93)
   d. Yes
   e. The population for the current study is breast cancer survivors, the scale was developed for that same population, test-retest reliability was confirmed since the instrument was used more than once. Cronbach's alpha coefficients were also provided as a measure of internal consistency and the scores were >0.70. Validity measures were not given in the article. The authors also discuss the methods used to maintain intervention fidelity during the study. Subjects in the study were randomly assigned to groups.
   f. The authors address threats to validity in the methods section, but not in the discussion, limitations, or recommendations sections.

Activity 6: Evidence-Based Practice Activity
First, this study would need to be put into context. It would need to be known what other studies were available in the same area. If a decision were being made based solely on the published reliability and validity information, it would not be considered a strong study.

To qualify this statement, there may be more information about the reliability and validity of the instruments. Some of it may have been cut to meet required article length. Some information is given, and what is presented is valuable and does lead to some confidence in the results—certainly more confidence than if they had been using several newly constructed instruments.

A final answer would be "it depends." Some questions would need to be asked and more listening would need to be done.

POSTTEST
1. Cronbach's alpha
2. Concurrent
3. Convergent
4. Content
5. Factor analysis
6. Interrater
7. Test-retest
8. Content
9. Convergent
10. Cronbach's alpha

CHAPTER 14

Activity 1
You will have your set of completed cards.

Activity 2
1. d
2. c
3. d
4. a
5. a, b, or c, depending on the tool used to measure satisfaction
6. a
7. b
8. d
9. a
10. c

Activity 3

Across
1. j Goofy's best friend
3. e Old abbreviation for mean
5. b Abbreviation for number of measures in a given data set (the measures may be individual people or some smaller piece of data such as blood pressure readings)
8. m Describes a set of data with a standard deviation of 3 when compared with a set of data with a standard deviation of 12
10. h Abbreviation for standard deviation
11. f Marks the "score" where 50% of the scores are higher and 50% are lower
12. c Measure of variation that shows the lowest and highest number in a data set

Down
1. l The values that occur most frequently in a data set
2. i 68% of the values in a normal distribution fall between ±1 of this statistic
4. d Can describe the height of a distribution
6. g Describes a distribution characterized by a tail
7. k Very unstable
9. a Measure of central tendency used with interval of ratio data

Activity 4

1. a. Pain duration
   b. Ordinal
2. a. DHHI
   b. SRAHP score
   c. Interval
3. a. Pain and race
   b. Nominal or ordinal; is a test of the difference between groups

Activity 5

1. Null hypothesis
2. Parametric statistics
3. Research hypothesis
4. Sampling error
5. Parameter; statistic
6. Correlation
7. Type II error; Type I error
8. Probability
9. Practical significance
10. Nonparametric statistics
11. Statistical significance

12. Research hypothesis; null hypothesis
13. c, b, a, e, d

Activity 6

1. $N = 12$
2. Nominal, ordinal, interval
3. 2.73
4. 2
5. 2
6. Limited sample size, $N = 12$; every score affects the mean

Activity 7

1. a. Yes
   b. Yes
   c. Yes
   d. Yes
2. All studies used descriptive statistics to describe certain characteristics of the sample (e.g., age, sex, ethnicity, marital status, income), except the study by Landreneau et al.—the descriptive data was included in a table but there was not a statistical analysis on the data.
3. Yes for all three studies with descriptive statistics.
4. The Horgas et al. study—because the purpose of the study was to describe pain, disability, and race using a specific model.
5. a. Yes
   b. Yes
   c. Yes
   d. No
6. a. Two-sample t-test, GEE marginal model, paired t-test
   b. Chi-square, t-tests, ANCOVA
   c. Chi-square, t-tests, SEM structural equation modeling
   d. Not applicable, because this is a qualitative study

Activity 8: Web-Based Activity

1. Four times more likely. Increased risk for males,16 to 19 years old, teens driving with teens, newly licensed teens, speeding, lower seat belt use.
2. 54% occur on these three days, and half of deaths occur between 3 PM and midnight.

Activity 9: Evidence-Based Practice Activity

School nurses should stop and consider how their actions could make a difference. They could check out the Web sites that are listed as references on the CDC site and look for recommendations of experts in the field. They could anticipate finding guidelines for ways of preventing risky driving in teen drivers. They could provide literature or education for parents of teens both before they are licensed and after. They may also need to devise a way to keep some data so there could be some evaluation of the steps they had taken (such as by asking someone in the local school of nursing to work with them on this task).

POSTTEST

1. This is a matter of personal preference and of probability. At clinic 1 you would have a longer average wait time, but 68% of the wait times would be from 30 to 50 minutes. At clinic 2, you may have a shorter wait sometimes but 68% of the wait times would be between 0 and 70 minutes.
2. The mean would provide information about the most common number of hospital gowns needed on your unit, but it is sensitive to outliers. The median could also be examined, but it is not clear if the hospital gown data has a normal distribution. Perhaps the best method would be to look at both the mean and median to determine the number of gowns for your unit. The mode may be useful, but again without knowing the distribution of the data, there is no way to know if the gown data has one mode or is bimodal. The mode would be less useful than the median and mean.

CHAPTER 15

Activity 1

1. R
2. D
3. R
4. D
5. R
6. R
7. R
8. D
9. D
10. D

Activity 2

1. Yes.
   * The table supplements and economizes the text. It would probably require about two pages of text to put all of the information in narrative form.
   * The title and headings are clear.
   * Does not repeat the information included in the text, it provides more detail than the text.
2. White.
3. Single in both groups.
4. Chi-squared test of difference in ethnic composition between the two groups.

Activity 3
Answers will vary from class to class.

Activity 4

1. a. There were 125 subjects in the experimental group, and $N = 132$ in the intervention group.
   b. SD was largest in the experimental group data from baseline to month 6. SD is a measure of variability.
   c. Standard deviation (SD) of 0.879. Within 0.879 (+/-) of the mean.
   d. This means that there is 1 chance in 1,000 that this result was due to chance. The smaller the p number, the more significant the result.
2. a. Overall quality of life and psychological well-being.
   b. Opinions may differ in the responses to this question.

Activity 5: Web-Based Activity

1. This answer will vary depending on when the search was conducted.
2. This answer will vary depending on when the search was conducted.

Activity 6: Evidence-Based Practice Activity
Answers will vary depending on when the Web site was accessed, and personal experience. The journal information and editorial policies are often found under "journal info" or a tab or link "for authors."

POSTTEST
1. b

2. T
3. d
4. F
5. b
6. c
7. F

CHAPTER 16

Please note that what follows are the results of one inspectional reading of the Meneses et al. article. You are not expected to agree with these findings. Some of you may agree, but many of you will not.

Systematic skimming: In reading the title, the fairly long abstract, the biographies, and the discussion, the following conclusions were made:
1. Yes, I am interested in oncology, so this population is one that would attract me.
2. The clinical area is related to an interest of mine.
3. I would proceed to superficial reading.

Superficial reading:
1. Remembered about the study:
   - Education was the treatment.
   - Intervention nurses were trained.
   - These data were based on a longitudinal study.
   - Quality of life was the driving theory.
   - This was a clinical study; it used experimental methods.
   - This would be Level II evidence.
   - The researchers ensured that the control group received the benefits of this psycho-educational program once the study was over. The study was approved by the IRB.
   - Instruments OK—used in other studies.
   - Data appeared to be OK.
   - The results were OK.
2. Conclusion: I would reread this study in greater detail. It contains some nuggets that could support some interests of mine. It would not be directly related to my research interests, but is interesting enough to be useful.
   Remember that the purpose of inspectional reading is to decide what to do about further reading of the study. What did you decide?

CHAPTER 17

Activity 1
1. Evidence-based practice is a broader term that includes the process of research utilization. Research utilization is focused on the application of research findings whereas evidence-based practice focused on the application of best-available evidence, which includes research findings in addition to nonresearch findings such as case reports and expert opinion.
2. a. the best-available evidence
   b. clinical expertise
   c. patient values

Activity 2
1. B
2. D
3. A
4. C
5. B
6. D

Activity 3
a. 5
b. 1
c. 7
d. 13
e. 2
f. 14
g. 6
h. 9
i. 11
j. 4
k. 8
l. 3
m. 12
n. 10

Activity 4
1. Conceptual; Decision
2. Problem-focused; Knowledge-focused
3. Patient, Population, or Problem; Intervention/ Treatment; Comparison Intervention/ Treatment; Outcome(s)
4. Stakeholder(s)

Activity 5: Web-based Activity
1. Addresses effective strategies for preventing and managing dental decay in the preschool child (Uribe, 2003, p. 4)

2. (P) Preschool children with and without dental decay in Scotland; (I) not applicable; (C) not applicable; (O) preventing and managing dental decay
3. Children with and without dental caries in Scotland (Uribe, 2003, p.16)
4. "Extensive panel of experts" (Uribe, 2003, p. 6); however, this is just a summary/abstract of the full guideline; if you were considering an evidence-based practice change you should retrieve the *full guideline* from http://www.sign.ac.uk/pdf/sign83.pdf, which states that the development group includes dental practitioners, health promotion professors
5. Not indicated; if you were considering an evidence-based practice change you would retrieve the full guideline from http://www.sign.ac.uk/pdf/sign83.pdf, which indicates that the guideline has information for parents and caregivers, including frequently asked questions (FAQ)
6. Dental teams working with community dental clinical as well as parents and crèche staff (p. 6)
7. Not indicated; also not indicated in *full guideline* from http://www.sign.ac.uk/pdf/sign83.pdf
8. Follows the SIGN methodology, which includes a search of EMBASE and MEDLINE from 1996 to 2003 and a range of Web sites for RCTs, meta-analyses, systematic reviews, observational studies; if you were considering an evidence-based practice change you should retrieve the SIGN methodology from http://www.sign.ac.uk/guidelines/fulltext/50/index.html
9. Not indicated; if you were considering an evidence-based practice change you would retrieve the *full guideline* from http://www.sign.ac.uk/pdf/sign83.pdf, which indicates that the full guideline was evaluated using methodological checklists before conclusions were considered as evidence; the *full guideline* also refers to the *SIGN 50: A Guideline Developer's Handbook* (http://www.sign.ac.uk/guidelines/fulltext/50/index.html), which you would want to retrieve if you were considering an evidence-based practice change.
10. Not indicated; if you were considering an evidence-based practice change you would retrieve the *full guideline* from http://www.sign.ac.uk/pdf/sign83.pdf, which indicates that the full guideline was evaluated using methodological checklists before conclusions were considered as evidence; the *full guideline* also refers the *SIGN 50: A Guideline Developer's Handbook* (http://www.sign.ac.uk/guidelines/fulltext/50/index.html), which you would want to retrieve if you were considering an evidence-based practice change.
11. Not indicated; if you were considering an evidence-based practice change you would retrieve the *full guideline* from http://www.sign.ac.uk/pdf/sign83.pdf, which indicates that the full guideline evaluated health benefits and risks, but not side effects, relative to certain interventions in the guideline.
12. Although the "Statements of Evidence" are presented, the recommendations are only linked to "Grades of Recommendations"; if you were considering an evidence-based practice change you would retrieve the *full guideline* from http://www.sign.ac.uk/pdf/sign83.pdf, which links the recommendations to both the "Levels of Evidence" and "Grades of Recommendations."
13. Not indicated; if you were considering an evidence-based practice change you would retrieve the *full guideline* from http://www.sign.ac.uk/pdf/sign83.pdf, which indicates that there has been consultation and peer review involved in reviewing the guideline.
14. Every 3 years (Uribe, 2004, p. 4).
15. The summary recommendations, which are linked to the "Grades of Recommendation," are specific and unambiguous.
16. No; usually evidence-based practice guidelines provide a clinical algorithm or flowchart that represents different options, which is most likely not applicable to this guidelines, "no clinical algorithm" (Uribe, 2003, p. 6).
17. The summary recommendations are provided and are easily identifiable; also if you were considering an evidence-based practice change you would retrieve the *full guideline* from http://www.sign.ac.uk/pdf/sign83.pdf, which indicates the summary recommendations on the last page.
18. Yes; however, in the article by Uribe (2003) it is not indicated; if you were considering an evidence-based practice change you should go to the SIGN Web site to retrieve all available information with the guideline; there is

a "Quick Reference Guide" that is available at http://www.sign.ac.uk/pdf/qrg83.pdf.

19. Not indicated; also not indicated in *full guideline* from http://www.sign.ac.uk/pdf/sign83.pdf.

20. Not indicated; if you were considering an evidence-based practice change you would retrieve the *full guideline* from http://www.sign.ac.uk/pdf/sign83.pdf, which indicates suggestions for "local implementation."

21. Not indicated; if you were considering an evidence-based practice change you would retrieve the *full guideline* from http://www.sign.ac.uk/pdf/sign83.pdf, which indicates suggestions for "key points for audit."

22. Not indicated; if you were considering an evidence-based practice change you would retrieve the *full guideline* from http://www.sign.ac.uk/pdf/sign83.pdf, which indicates the SIGN editorial groups, which gives an idea of some of the SIGN members but not all.

23. Not indicated; if you were considering an evidence-based practice change you would retrieve the *full guideline* from http://www.sign.ac.uk/pdf/sign83.pdf, which indicates suggestions that declarations of interest were made by all members of the guideline development group.

Activity 6

National Guideline Clearinghouse (http://www.guideline.gov); American Pain Society (http://www.ampainsoc.org); Oncology Nursing Society (http://www.ons.org); the American Association of Critical-Care Nurses (http://www.aacn.org); Registered Nurses Association of Ontario (http://www.rnao.org); National Institute for Health and Clinical Excellence (http://www.nice.org.uk); the Association for Women's Health, Obstetrics, and Neonatal Nursing (http://www.awhonn.org); the Gerontological Nursing Interventions Research Center (http://www.nursing.uiowa.edu/excellence/nursing_interventions/index.htm); the American Thoracic Society (http://www.thoracic.org).

Activity 7

1. Y
2. N
3. Y
4. Y
5. N
6. Y

Activity 8

1. b
2. a. Revision of professional roles
   b. Multidisciplinary teams
   c. Integrated care services
   d. Interventions aimed at knowledge management
   e. Quality management
3. c
4. a
5. Opinion leaders; change champions, core groups; academic detailing

POSTTEST

1. Pediatric cardiology on 14 diagnosis groups
2. "Appointed CPG coordinator and the collaboration of all members of the healthcare team. The CPG steering group consists of expert clinicians, including the Vice President of Cardiovascular Critical Care Services, attending cardiologists, anesthesiologists and surgeons, clinical coordinators, nurse practitioners, staff nurses, patient care coordinator, respiratory therapists, nutritionist, and social worker" (Poppleton, Moynihan, & Hickey, 2003, p. 76).
3. It appears that all members of the team could be considered stakeholders; key stakeholders not represented could include patients (if applicable due to age), patients' families, senior hospital leadership (both medical and nursing).
4. Not indicated
5. Not indicated
6. Not indicated
7. Not indicated; not indicated
8. To a degree; however recommendations are missing an indication to the evidence to support the recommendations and the grade of the evidence
9. Not indicated
10. Detailed methodology for how patient data would be collected, including an excerpt from a sample clinical guideline and a variance tracking sheet for a sample clinical guideline
11. Yes; yes, "the CPG Program has been a successful strategy in a continual effort to provide cost effective care without compromising quality" (Poppleton et al., 2003, p. 83), the authors report several positive outcomes
12. CPG coordinator could be considered both "Change Champion" (due to clinical expertise

qualities) and "Opinion Leader" (due to technological qualities) both of which encompass EBP expertise; didactic education (education during orientation and when new CPGs are introduced)

CHAPTER 18

Activity 1

1. a. P—older adults
    b. I—measures of adiposity
    c. C—cardiorespiratory fitness*
    d. O—mortality*
    e. P or C/H (this study is a prognosis study)
        *Note: In nontherapy studies, there may be more than one intervention or comparison, or an intervention without comparison.
2. a. P—patients with diabetic foot ulcers
    b. I—negative pressure wound therapy (NPWT) using vacuum-assisted closure
    c. C—advanced moist wound therapy (AMWT)
    d. O—wound healing
    e. Therapy
3. a. P—adolescent clinical patients
    b. I—CRAFFT
    c. C—none*
    d. O—screening for substance abuse
    e. Diagnosis
        *Note: In nontherapy studies, there may be more than one intervention or comparison, or an intervention without comparison
4. a. P—children
    b. I—residential exposure to power line magnetic fields
    c. C—none
    d. O—ALL
    e. C/H
        *Note: In nontherapy studies, there may be more than one intervention or comparison, or an intervention without comparison.

Activity 2

1. Therapy; Prognosis; Causation; Review; Qualitative
2. None
3. Clinical Trial; Meta-Analysis; Practice Guideline; Randomized Controlled Trial

4. Etiology; Diagnosis; Therapy; Prognosis; Clinical Predication Guides
5. PUBMED (Medline)—"Clinical Queries"

Activity 3

1. P—adolescents and adults with type 2 diabetes in Miami; I—unknown; C—usual care; O—hemoglobin $A_{1C} < 7.0\%$.
2. P—adults age 18 to 89 with type 2 diabetes in Minnesota; I—TRANSLATE; C—usual care; O—hemoglobin $A_{1C} < 7.0\%$.
3. There would be concern that the target population (adolescents and adults with type 2 diabetes) could be different than the study population (adults age 18 to 89); in addition, there could be differences inherent to the location of the target population (Miami) versus the study population (Minnesota).
4. Yes; the study was unblinded.
5. The percentage of patients who achieved a hemoglobin $A_{1C} < 7.0\%$ (and thus percentage of patients not achieving a hemoglobin $A_{1C} < 7.0\%$); discrete/dichotomous.
6. "1.0." Note: The null value varies depending on the outcome; for a continuous outcome variable the null value would be "0.0."
7. Patients in the intervention group were 12% more likely to achieve hemoglobin $A_{1C} < 7.0\%$ than those in the control group. In order for 1 patient to benefit, 20 patients need to receive the intervention.
8. RBI is statistically significant because the CI does not include 1.0 (the null value); the NNT is statistically significant because the CI does not include 1.0 (the null value).
9. Although an average of 20 patients would need to be receive the intervention in order for 1 patient to benefit, it could be as low at 14 to as high as 35 patients (which is a wide range) who would need to receive the intervention in order for one patient to benefit. Depending on implementation issues (i.e., cost, time, manpower) it may not be clinically significant to have to provide the intervention to 35 patients for just 1 patient to benefit.
10. Although patients in the intervention group were significantly more likely to achieve hemoglobin $A_{1C} < 7.0\%$ statistically, given that (a) the population in the study may differ from that of the clinical situation (target population) and that (b) clinical significance may be questionable, applying the results of

the study to the target population should be done with caution, and it would not be likely that an evidence-based practice change would be made based on this one study.

Activity 4

1. P—U.S. teenage girls; I—not applicable; C—not applicable; O—eating disorders
2. There would be concern that the difference in geographic locations of the target population (California) and study population (Spain) would be significantly different even though the clinical situation PICO question and study question are similar.
3. Causation because the clinical situation and study are about determining whether one thing is related to another; based on the study design (cohort study) you would select the CASP Tool for Cohort Studies.
4. a. Discrete/dichotomous
   b. Discrete/dichotomous
   c. Discrete/dichotomous
   d. Discrete/dichotomous
5. Teenage girls whose parents were not married, who ate alone, who read girls' magazines more than once per week, and who listened to the radio for more than 1 hour per day were at increased odds for developing an eating disorder; all of these variables (except for "reading girls' magazines more than once per week") were statistically significantly associated with an increase in odds for developing an eating disorder; the null value is "1.0"; the CI for the variables of "parents' marital status", "eating alone", and "listening to the radio" do not include "1.0," indicating that these results are statistically significant, whereas the CI for the "reading girls' magazines more than once per week" (0.91 to 2.2) includes "1.0," indicating that it is not statistically significant.
6. Although results of this study reflect a population of teenage girls from Spain, it is possible that there may be credibility in applying the

evidence to the current clinical situation. Although an evidence-based practice change may not be warranted by this one study, a further review, critical appraisal, and synthesis of the evidence could lead to changes in screening teenage girls for eating disorders in the target population.

POSTTEST

1. False; an experimental or quasi-experimental study design is usually used for the therapy category of clinical concern used by clinicians; causation/harm studies typically use nonexperimental (longitudinal or retrospective) study designs
2. True
3. True
4. False; a meta-analysis is a quantitative approach to a systematic review that can only be performed if "combining" the results of the individual studies is reasonable (usually if the results of the individual studies are homogeneous or similar from study to study)
5. False; *sensitivity* is the proportion of those with the disease who test positive and *specificity* is the proportion of those without the disease who test negative
6. False; the CI provides the reader information about both the statistical and clinical significance of the findings; although findings may be statistically significant, the clinician must apply the "low" and "high" end of the confidence levels to determine clinical significance
7. True
8. True
9. True
10. False; *likelihood ratio* is a term used to describe the number that expresses the sensitivity, specificity, PPV, NPV, and prevalence for diagnosis clinical category questions

Notes

Notes

Notes

Notes